Sirtfood Diet

Complete Guide for A Quick Weight Loss and Restoring Health. Burn Fat Activating Your "Skinny Gene" with Easy and Delicious Recipes

By

Harry S. Parker

Disclaimer Notice

Please note that the information contained in this document is for educational and entertainment purposes only. All effort has been made to present accurate, up-to-date, reliable, complete information. No warranties of any kind are declared or implied. Readers acknowledge that the author is not engaging in the rendering of legal, financial, medical, or professional advice. The content of this book was gathered from various sources. Please consult a licensed professional before attempting any of the techniques discussed in this book.

By reading this document, the reader agrees that under no circumstances is the author responsible for any losses, direct or indirect, which are incurred as a result of the use of the information contained within this document, including, but not limited to errors, omissions, and inaccuracies.

Table of Contents

Introduction

I want to thank and congratulate you for downloading this book, *"**Sirtfood Diet**."*

Of the many people to adopt this year's popularized diets, fewer than one percent will gain significant weight loss. Not only are they failing to make a difference in the bulge war, but they're doing nothing to stem the wave of chronic disease that has engulfed modern society.

When we crop on calories, this causes an energy shortage that stimulates what's referred to as the "skinny gene," causing a torrent of positive change. It puts the body in a quiet survival mode where fat is prevented from being processed, and expected growth processes are placed on hold.

Instead, the body turns its attention to burning up its fat stores and flipping on its powerful housekeeping genes that fix and rejuvenate our cells, effectively giving them a spring clean. The upshot is weight loss and heightened disease resistance.

Yet, cutting calories, as many dieters know, comes at a price. Reducing energy intake in the short-term causes hunger, irritability, fatigue, and muscle loss. Long-term restriction on calories causes our metabolism to stagnate. This fact is often the collapse of all calorie-restrictive diets and paves the way for a piling the weight back on. For these reasons, 99 percent of dieters are doomed to long-term failure.

All this led us to ask an enormous question: is it possible to somehow activate our thin gene, with all the wonderful benefits - that carry all those disadvantages - without having an extreme calorie limit?

Enter Sirtfoods, a set of newly discovered wonder-foods. Sirtfoods are particularly rich in certain nutrients, which will become skinny genes in our bodies, acting as a calorie restriction does. These genes are called sirtuins.

This book looks at the Sirtfood diet in some detail and is meant to answer many of the foremost essential questions the Sirtfood diet raises. Such as:

What is Sirtfood?

What are Sirtuins?

Ultimately, you'll face the foremost important question of all:

Who should try the Sirtfood diet?

The information in these pages is meant to help you discover the answers to those questions.

In this book, you'll also find many various recipes: Breakfast, Fluids, Main Meals, Salads, Snacks, Juices, Cocktails and Desserts. Because of the different recipes, there are delicious dishes for everybody.

Let's proceed!

The Basics of the Sirtfood Diet

This diet relies on research sirtuins (SIRTs), a group of seven proteins utilized from the human anatomy, that have been proven to moderate inflammation, metabolism, and increase life expectancy.

"Sirtfoods" are foods with the ability to increase the amount of those proteins in the body.

What Is the Sirtfood Diet?

The diet blends sirtfoods and calorie limitation, causing the body to produce an increased amount of sirtuins.

This Sirtfood Diet book comprises meal plans and recipes to follow along; however, there are many other Sirtfood Diet recipe books out there.

The diet's founders claim that a Sirtfood Diet can cause accelerated weight loss while maintaining muscle mass and protecting you from chronic illness.

Once you finish the dietary plan, you're invited to add sirtfoods and the diet's signature green juice to your regular diet.

There are no evident sign that the Sirtfood diet causes increased weight loss than a calorie-restricted diet regime.

Although various foods have beneficial properties, there are yet to be any long-term human studies to determine if eating a diet filled with sirtfoods has any concrete health benefits.

Nonetheless, the Sirtfood Diet publication's pilot study's outcomes were as follows:

After one week of following the diet and working out each day, the participants lost almost 5 pounds (3.2 kg) and claimed that they even gained some muscle tissue.

Yet, these outcomes are hardly surprising. Restricting your calorie intake to 1000 calories while exercising throughout the same period will almost always trigger weight loss.

This sort of fast fat reduction is not suitable for the long-term.

When your body is energy-deprived, it uses your emergency energy stores of glycogen while burning muscle and fat.

Each molecule of glycogen necessitates 3-4 atoms of water. Whenever your body uses glycogen, it removes water.

In the first week of an extreme calorie deficit, almost one-fifth of these weight loss is from fat, whereas one other two-thirds stems from water, glycogen, and muscle.

When your calories increase, the body replenishes its glycogen stores and you regain the lost weight.

Unfortunately, such a calorie deficit can cause the body to scale back its metabolism, meaning you require fewer calories per day.

A diet may help you lose a few pounds initially but once you finish dieting you are likely to put on the lost weight.

Three weeks could be long enough to have some measurable long-term effects for preventing illness.

Alternatively, adding sirtfoods to a routine diet might just be an incredible idea in the long term. You could finish your diet and start eating sirtfoods today.

History of the Sirt Diet

One way to gauge a diet plan is to look at it in the context of others. Are the ideas new and revolutionary? Or, are they just an old method with a bit of spin on them? Maybe an old notion is bad only because it's been around for a while? Is a new idea terrible because it hasn't?

Most modern recipes would appear strange to inhabitants of the traditional world as many of the foods readily available to us – tomatoes, potatoes, sugar, for instance, were unknown. Even an egg, for example, wasn't relatively easy to get hold of until the domestication of chickens, which didn't happen until 500 B.C.E.

It's fair to mention that the typical person was more concerned by hunger than by their weight. But by the time of the traditional Greeks, things had changed. Anyone who aspired to be beautiful had to have the body to show for it, and since nakedness wasn't a no-no for the traditional Greeks and if they wanted to talk the talk they also had to be able to walk the walk.

One significant difference between then and now was the perfect image of beauty: lithe and muscular. This may be very similar to today, but it was almost exclusively male. The Greeks didn't think women were on an equivalent level to men, physically, mentally or emotionally.

The Roman Empire, famous for self-indulgence, ate food similar to modern Italian cuisine with a couple of exceptions like tomatoes, capsicum, spinach, and egg-plant that was yet to be imported from the east. The traditional Romans ate meat which could be seen as strange to us, such as dormice and snails. Fish was more common at meals than meat. The pattern of today's meals – appetizer, main course, and dessert – was set around the time of the Republic and has remained ever since with one major exception: the meals in ancient Rome took far longer than ours! On just one occasion, historians believed Romans vomited between courses to make room for more food. This has been suggested to have been a misinterpretation.

One of the famous historical diets was that of William The Conqueror. Embarrassed by being unable to mount his horse, William selected a diet of liquid alcohol; after all, it meant no food. Sadly, the diet didn't work too well, and when poor William subsequently died from an infection, he was so large he had to be pressed into his coffin, where, sadly, his intestines burst.

By the time of the Renaissance, women spent their lives trussed in corsets. In an age long before zippers (or even buttons), weight gain could sometimes be hidden by lacing corsets tighter or the dress loosely, but the pressure to remain slim was already on. Many ladies developed sores from tightly laced corsets and died when the sores became infected. The perfect woman of the time was somewhat rounder than today, as are often seen in Renaissance statuary and paintings.

What Are Sirtuins

Sirtuins, shortened to SIRT, are among the family of proteins that function to manage cellular health, including homeostasis. Homeostasis is the body's process that maintains stability and adjusts to best suit the surrounding conditions.

The SIRT protein family has seven members (SIRT1-7). SIR2 yeast silent information regulator is that the SIRT protein family's founding member controls chromatin, DNA recombination, and organic phenomenon. Among the seven mammalian SIRTs, SIRT1, SIRT2, and SIRT3 have the power to deacetylase. Other remaining SIRTs (SIRT4, SIRT5, SIRT6, and SIRT7) possess a weak or no detectable deacetylates activity.

SIRT1-7 differ in function and cellular localization. SIRT1 is found in the cytosol and nucleus, where it performs its function for cellular life. It's involved in glucose metabolism, neurodegeneration, differentiation, control of organic phenomenon, aging, necrobiosis, and tumorigenesis. SIRT2, located in the cytosol, helps catalyze Alpha tubulin's deacetylation (Lys40), H31ys56, FOXO1, H41ys16, and FOXO3a.

It's involved in organic phenomenon regulation, tubulin acetylation, tubulin acetylation, cell cycle regulation, DNA damage response, cancer, neurodegeneration.

SIRT3 location in mitochondria inner membrane with substrates of long-chain acyl-CoA dehydrogenase

(LCDA), acetyl-CoA synthetase 2 (ACS2), 2,3-hydroxy-3-methyl-glutaryl CoA synthetase 2 (HMGCS2), ornithine transcarbamoylase transferase (OTC), glutamate dehydrogenase (GDH), Cycle-Philip D, SOD 2(SOD2), isocitrate dehydrogenase 2 (IDH2), numerous components of the mitochondria respiratory chain complexes also as Ku70.

It's liable for mitochondria ATP production, carboxylic acid oxidation, and mitochondrial protein regulation. Also, it controls caloric restriction and cellular response to oxidative stress through the activation of SOD2 and IDH2, which can, in turn, reduce oxidized reactive oxygen species (ROS) and glutathione. It also involved in tumor suppression and necrobiosis, thereby influencing genomic stability positively. SIRT4 is found in the Mitochondrial Matrix.

It's involved in ADP-ribosylation and GHD inhibition by utilizing NAD+. SIRT5, also localized in the mitochondrial Matrix, contains an NAD+ dependent decarboxylase and desuccinylase activity on CPS1. SIRT6, functioning as deacetylase, and ADPribosyltransferase is essential telomeric functions, metabolism hemostasis, DNA repair, genome stability.

SIRT7 is a predominantly nucleolar protein that regulates gene transcription by interacting with RNA polymerase 1. SIRT7 has high selectivity for the H31ys18 and also features an NAD+ dependent deacetylase. When SIRT7 gets deacetylated, we'd like to repress genes involved in cellular Anchorage and get in touch with inhibition, thereby favoring the malignant phenotype tumor cells.

The Sirtfood Science

The sirtfood diet can't be classified as low-carb or low-fat. This diet is different from its many predecessors, it has similar features, it advocates for the ingestion of fresh, plant-based foods. As the name implies, it is often based on a sirtuin based diet. What are sirtuins? Why have you ever never heard about them before?

There are seven sirtuin proteins – SIRT-1 to SIRT-71. They are found throughout your cells and the cells of every animal on earth. Sirtuins are found in almost every living organism and practically every part of the cell and control what goes on.

Supplement company, Elysium Health, likens the body's cells to an office, with sirtuins acting as the CEO, helping the cells react to internal and external changes. They govern what's done when it's done, and who does it.

Of the seven sirtuins, one works in your cell's cytoplasm, three in the cell's mitochondria, and another in the cell's nucleus. They have a number of jobs to perform, but mostly they remove acetyl groups from other proteins. These acetyl groups signal that the protein they're attached to is out there to perform its function. Sirtuins remove the available flag and obtain the protein.

Sirtuins sound pretty crucial to your body's normal function, so why is it that you do never heard of them before?

The first sirtuin to be discovered was SIR2, a gene found in the 1970s that controlled fruit flies' power to mate. It wasn't until the 1990s that scientists discovered other, similar proteins in almost every sort of life. Every organism had a particular number of sirtuins – bacteria has one, and yeast has five.

Experiments on mice show they need an equivalent number as humans, seven.

Sirtuins are shown to prolong life in yeast and mice. There is, so far, no evidence of an equivalent effect in the citizenry. However, these sirtuins are present in almost every sort of life. Many scientists are hopeful that if organisms as far apart as yeast and mice can see an equivalent effect from sirtuin activation, this might also reach humans.

Our bodies need another substance called nicotinamide adenine dinucleotide for cells to function properly, in addition to sirtuins. Elysium (see above) likens this substance to the cash a corporation must have to keep operating. Like the CEO, a sirtuin can only keep the corporate side working properly if the income is sufficient. NAD+ was first discovered in 1906. You get your supply of NAD+ from your diet by eating foods made up of the building blocks of NAD+.

Fun Facts About Sirtuins:

— Mice engineered to possess high levels of SIRT-1 are both more active and leaner than normal. In contrast, mice that lack SIRT-1 altogether are fatter and more susceptible to various metabolic conditions.

— Add the very fact that levels of SIRT-1 are much lower in obese people than in those of a "healthy" weight, and the case for the importance of sirtuins in weight loss becomes compelling.

— By making a permanent change to your diet and adding the simplest sirtfoods to your eating plan, the authors of their food diet believe everyone can improve their health, without losing muscle mass.

The Sirtfood for Weight Loss

Research conducted by Aidan Goggins and Glen Martin showed that 7 pounds of weight were lost on average in seven days on the Sirt food diet after accounting for muscle gain. Sirtuins' diet has not only promised weight loss but increased healthiness. A rise in the level of body sirtuins has been proven to cause weight loss. The simplest way of accelerating body leptin remains through fasting and exercise. Also, one of the simplest forms of enhancing body sirtuins is by consumption of sirtuin foods. All of these components will affect body metabolism, which we'll discuss in the next chapter.

Furthermore, hypothalamic SIRT1 has been proven to assist weight loss. The hypothalamus is the central weight and energy balance controller. It modulates energy intake and energy consumption by neural inputs from the periphery and direct humor inputs, which senses the body's energy status. An adipokine, leptin, is one of the factors that signal that sufficient energy is stored on the periphery. Leptin plasma levels are favorable for adiposity, suppressing energy intake, and stimulating energy spending. A protracted increase in the level of plasma leptin in obese can cause leptin resistance. Leptin resistance, in turn, can affect the hypothalamus from having access to leptin, which also reduces leptin signals transduction in the hypothalamic neurons. Reduced peripheral energy-sensing by leptin can cause a positive energy balance and incremental weight gain and adiposity improvements, further exacerbating leptin resistance. Leptin resistance causes a rise in adiposity. Similar observations occur in central insulin resistance. Therefore, the development of humoral factors in the hypothalamus can prevent progressive weight gains, especially among middle-aged individuals. SIRT1 may be a protein deacetylase, NAD+ dependent, with many substrates, like transcription factors, histones, co-factors, and various enzymes. SIRT1 improves the sensitivity to leptin and insulin by decreasing several molecules that impair leptin and insulin signals' transduction. The hypothalamic SIRT1 and NAD+ levels decrease with age. An increase in the level of SIRT1 has been shown to enhance kept in level in mice, then prevents age-related weight gain. By controlling the loss of age-dependent SIRT1 hypothalamus role, there'll be a lift in the activity of humoral factors in the hypothalamus and, therefore, the central energy balance control.

Sirtfood for Building Muscle

Sirtuins are a group of proteins with different effects. Sirt-1 is the protein liable for causing the body to burn fat instead of muscle for energy, which is a miracle for weight loss. Another useful aspect of Sirt-1 is its ability to enhance striated muscle.

Skeletal muscle is all the muscles you voluntarily control, like your limbs' muscles, back, shoulders, etc.

There are two other types; the heart muscle is what the guts are made of, while the smooth muscle is your involuntary muscles – which incorporates muscles around your blood vessels, face, and various parts of organs and other tissues.

Skeletal muscle is separated into two different groups, the blandly named type-1 and type-2. Type 1 muscle is significant at continued, sustained activity, whereas type-2 is significant at short, intense periods of activity. So, for instance, you'd predominantly use type-1 muscles for jogging but type-2 muscles for sprinting.

Sirt-1 protects the type-1 muscles, but not the type-2, which remains weakened for energy. Therefore, holistic muscle mass drops when fasting, albeit type-1 striated muscle mass increases.

Sirt-1 also influences how the muscles work. Sirt-1 is produced by the muscle cells, but the power to supply Sirt-1 decreases because of the muscle ages. As a result, muscle is harder to create as you age and doesn't grow as fast in response to exercise. A scarcity of Sirt-1 also causes the muscles to become bored quickly and gradually decline over time.

When you start to think about these effects of Sirt-1, you'll begin to make an image about why fasting helps keep the body supple. Fasting releases Sirt-1, which successively helps striated muscle grow and stay in good condition. Sirt-1 is additionally released by consuming sirtuin activators, giving the sirtfood diet its muscle retaining power.

Who Should Try Sirtfood Diet?

The SirtFood Diet is suitable for people who:

- — Are overweight or obese

- — Want to take care of his/her weight

- — Needs to have a "detox" and flush away the toxins from the body

- — Did not get the desired results from other dieting techniques

- — Want to lose weight while building muscle

- — Want a healthier lifestyle

Health Risks for Overweight and Obesity

— Type 2 Diabetes: This disease occurs when the blood glucose level becomes above the traditional. Consistent with studies, about 80% of people who have Type 2 diabetes are overweight. What makes diabetes a killer disease is that it's a severe explanation for stroke, a heart condition, kidney diseases, amputation, and even blindness.

— Sleep Apnea: This often is when a private pause in breathing while sleeping. Being overweight or obese may be a risk factor. Why? Usually, this is due to the fats stored in the neck area, making the air pathway smaller. Additionally, the fat could also cause inflammation. Apnea shouldn't be taken lightly because it also can end in coronary failure.

— High vital sign: Also referred to as hypertension, this condition refers to a state when your systolic vital sign (usually above 140) is consistently above your diastolic vital sign (usually about 90). How does being overweight cause you to high risk for hypertension? Generally, a bigger body size will increase your vital sign so that your heart will need to work harder to supply the necessary supply of blood to all or any cells. Additionally, your excess body fats can damage your kidneys (your kidney helps your body regulate blood pressure). A high vital sign may result in renal failure, heart diseases, and stroke.

— Fatty Liver Disease - this often is when there's a build-up of fat around the liver, which may cause damage.

— Reproductive issues: Menstrual issues and ultimately, infertility are a number of the problems experienced by overweight women.

— Cancer: If you're obese or overweight, then the danger of acquiring cancer of the breast, gallbladder, colon, and endometrial increases.

These are just some of the diseases related to being overweight, not to mention the additional weight's social, emotional, and psychological impact.

It stresses the importance of finding the right "strategy" to lose those excess pounds. And for that we have the right solution —the Sirtfood diet.

Are you conversant in these scenarios?

You know that you simply have overindulged in the vacations, but as you weigh yourself, you literally would want to shave all the additional pounds because you probably did not expect to possess gained that much weight!

There is an upcoming wedding event, and you would like to lose those extra pounds to suit you into your gown/suit. There's no way that you only are getting to lose that much weight in 2 months!

You know that you simply are overweight and just plain unhealthy. You do already tried a variety of diets but to no avail. Either you feel that those diets are too restrictive, there's an adverse health effect, and therefore the diet is just too expensive to take care of. Speaking of maintenance, you have a tough time keeping off the small weight that you have managed to lose!

You are getting older, and you begin to note that apart from having a tough time handling hangovers and late-night parties, losing and maintaining weight isn't as easy as it used to be. You're not an enormous fan of eliminating numerous food groups and doing rigorous exercise.

You have probably heard these scenarios several times before, and you've probably experienced one or two. Being overweight or obese is one of the most significant health problems in the world. Consistent with the World Health Organization (WHO), being overweight is when your BMI is adequate to or greater than 25 while being obese is when your BMI is equal to or greater than 30. (You can check your BMI here.)

In the 2014 data from WHO, worldwide obesity has doubled since 1980, and 1.9 billion adults are overweight. It may be safe to conclude that after two years that that number has already increased significantly.

Health experts agree that this is an alarming rate, but the great news is, obesity or having excess weight is preventable and reversible.

As you'll notice, most of those scenarios are focused on the aesthetics—looking good and feeling more confident about your body, but what I wish to stress is that the ill-effects of each extra bulge or pound that we feature. The possible health illnesses related to being overweight are why you would like to undertake the revolutionary Sirtfood Diet.

Health Benefits of Sirtfood Diet

It's no accident that some individuals with long lifespan and healthiest populations in the world eat diets rich in these sirtuin-activating foods; examples are those in the Mediterranean and parts of Asia. The Mediterranean diet includes polyphenol-rich fruits, veggies, vegetable oil, including wine. The Asian diet is rich in isoflavones present in soya beans and epigallactins from tea.

Including several of those health developing foods into your diet is proportionately comfortable. They will be included in many diets and even compound to make super-sirt meals!

Discussed below are several benefits of the sirtfood diet and also its pros and cons.

Sirtfoods Fight Fat

When starting a diet, everybody expects to lose weight and feel great. However, you would like to have the right expectations from the start.

The problem with most diets is that you'll revisit your unhealthy eating habits as soon as you quit them, and you'll put on the weight you have lost. The critical challenge is to take care of your weight if you're satisfied with the weight loss thus far.

This means that you need to stick to your diet, regardless. When it comes to the fat-burning process, the foremost powerful sirtuin is SIRT1. Because it seems, bodies with a better concentration of SIRT1 are leaner and have a more active metabolism. This fact was noticed in mice and may be readily applicable to humans. In other words, this specific sirtuin activates the thin gene, capable of controlling your weight.

However, the advantages of SIRT1 don't stop there. It fights against PPAR-y (peroxisome proliferator-activated receptor-y), a group of nuclear receptor proteins liable for the fat-gain process. These receptors simply trigger the genes required to synthesize and store fat. To stop this from happening, PPAR-y must be stopped. Well, this often is what SIRT1 does. It wipes out the assembly and storage of fat and accelerates your metabolism so your body can remove the surplus fat. This can't be avoided by creating mitochondria (the energy factories from each of our cells). In other words, the more mitochondria you have (energy), the more fat you'll burn because it can allow you to interact in several physical fat-burning activities.

There are two sorts of fat storages: white fat (WAT) and brown fat (BAT). The primary one is typically related to weight gain fat, but the other behaves differently, and it's even beneficial. This tissue is understood for producing energy in the form of heat. The WAT is the one you would like to focus on, as this is often the tissue that encourages fat accumulation, making us overweight or maybe obese. This is where sirtuins can perform a bit of magic, as they will make white fat possess comparable properties to the brown one. This is what's called "the browning effect." In plain words, the fat from the WAT is going to be mobilized for disposal.

But wait, there's more! Sirtuins don't just encourage fat to disappear; it also features a very positive effect on insulin itself. As you almost certainly know, weight gain is additionally related to increased levels of insulin. SIRT1 can be very helpful when it involves lowering insulin resistance. Moreover, it encourages the discharge of thyroid hormones, so it plays an important role in speeding up your metabolism and burning fat.

Most overweight and obese people are hooked to carbs and processed food, named caloric bombs but have low nutritional value. The ingredients of a sirtfood diet can easily reverse leptin resistance. It makes sure that leptins signal your brain about the important level of nutrient intake. Moreover, people are not experiencing hunger when trying this diet (unlike any fasting program). Indeed, everything comes right down to your brain, but when the right information reaches your brain (leptins), you do away a higher chance of controlling your appetite.

Build Muscle Mass

When people mention that they need to lose weight, they're talking about losing fat, not muscle. Fat is lighter than muscle, but we all want to possess an optimal BMI, right? There's a myth stating that you simply need a particular amount of proteins to preserve your muscle mass. Well, that's not entirely true. In the case of fasting, the expansion hormone reaches incredibly high levels after 72 hours of pure fasting, so you'll preserve and even increase your muscle mass through calorie deprivation. It's not healthy to get on a long period of fasting, but what if you found the right ingredients to eat and have equivalent benefits.

This meal plan is meant to save lots of your muscles and only obviate what you hate most: the unaesthetic fat tissue makes you feel heavy and not agile. Therefore, how can you reduce your fat and keep your existing muscles? This is what the sirtfood diet is aiming for and it is doing an excellent job. Do you know why? Because it makes your body run on fats as an energy source. You're not overfeeding yourself with glucose; instead, you have very balanced diet that burn fats.

Moreover, it doesn't attack your muscle mass, and once you have more muscles, you'll burn more energy. The more energy you burn, the more fat you burn. Muscles are built through workouts. You merely can't just eat food, do nothing, and expect to possess strength. Otherwise, we would all eat like hell and still have muscles. As any bodybuilder would tell you: "No pain, no gain."

However, the food must create the right environment to build muscle mass or preserve it, which is what this diet is doing. After all, muscles are essential for your mobility, and they prevent chronic diseases like osteoporosis or diabetes from happening. Believe it or not, but forces can even have a psychological advantage, as they're known to fight against depression. Yep, you'll feel great about yourself once you have a sporty look.

SIRT1 can preserve the muscle mass even once you are browsing fasting, and it can even increase your striated muscle mass. Muscles are composed of several cells, including the satellite cell, activated when the muscles are broken or stressed. If you're performing some weight training, basically applying stress to the muscle, your muscles will get bigger thanks to the satellite cell. However, the satellite cell can only be triggered by SIRT1; otherwise, your muscles won't grow, develop, or regenerate properly.

Just to enforce the importance of sirtuins, especially SIRT1, keep in mind that without them, muscles are subject to inflammation and fatigue. Muscles are aging without the activity of sirtuins. Therefore, to function correctly, muscles need SIRT1. Muscles don't recover in time, a bit like wine does. Bear in mind that the consequences of muscle aging can start at the age of 25. By the time you reach 40, you have already lost 10 percent of your muscle mass, and once you are in your 70s, you do already lost 40 percent of your muscle mass. However, this will be prevented and reversed through the activity of sirtuins. Hence, they will easily be considered as regulators of muscle prevention and growth.

Sirtfoods Fight Diseases

Medicine is progressing, but this doesn't mean that people are becoming healthier. It's quite the opposite. Around 70 percent of the deaths nowadays are caused by chronic diseases. This is shocking, but the cause is often traced to the food we eat. Medicine is advancing because it's challenged, but you'd be surprised that the antidote to most of our diseases is healthy food. Processed food causes these issues, but healthy food can make it right.

The modern-day eating habits and lifestyle encourage the buildup of fats and toxins (fat tissue protects the toxins) and blood glucose and insulin level. This is where the difficulty starts, from a comfortable prediabetes condition to more severe diseases (it can eventually cause cancer). However, the antidote to many of those issues lies hidden in ourselves. As you already know, all bodies possess sirtuin genes, and activating them is crucial to burn fat and create a healthier and leaner body.

As it seems, the advantages of sirtuins activity extend way beyond the fat-burning process. Whether we love it or not, the shortage of sirtuins is often related to many diseases and medical conditions. Naturally, activating sirtuins will have the other effect. For instance, sirtuins can improve your heart health by protecting your heart's muscle cells and improving the guts muscle's function. But that's not all. Sirtuins can play a severe role in enhancing your arteries' function, controlling cholesterol levels, and preventing atherosclerosis.

By now, you're conversant in the consequences of fasting and an LCHF diet on the insulin level, and you're probably wondering what sirtuins can neutralize this case. If you're affected by diabetes, you should know that activating sirtuins will make insulin work more effectively to properly do its job (regulating the blood glucose level). SIRT1 works perfectly with metformin (one of the foremost powerful antidiabetic drugs). Because it seems, pharmaceutical companies are adding sirtuin activators to metformin treatments. These studies were conducted on animals, and therefore the results were simply excellent. It had been noticed that an 83 percent reduction of the metformin dose is required to realize equivalent effects.

Other diets or programs are bragging about their effects on neurodegenerative diseases, like Alzheimer's disease. Well, let's believe what sirtuins do! They send a message to the brain, helping it make the right decisions when it involves appetite suppression. This consists of enhancing the brain's communication signals, improving cognitive function, and lowering brain inflammation. Sirtuin activation stops the tau protein aggregation and amyloid β production, a number of the most dangerous things in Alzheimer's patients' brains.

The benefits of sirtuins expand to bones also, as they encourage the assembly of osteoblast cells (the ones liable for strengthening your bones) and increase their survival. In other words, sirtuin activation is essential for overall bone health.

We all know that the food we eat today can even cause cancer, as we eat small portions of poison. Diets are claiming that they represent the cure for cancer in an incipient make, but at the instant, we can't say this about sirtfoods, as there are still many studies to be done on this subject. However, it's fair to mention those people that mostly eat sirtfoods have rock bottom cancer rates.

Losing weight is just not enough nowadays because the diet you follow must have many health benefits as well; otherwise, you can't stick with it at the end of the day. Therefore, you would like to ascertain the larger picture and not specialize in losing tons of pounds in a concise amount of your time. Radical diets usually accompany side effects, but if you discover a hotel plan that works for you regarding weight loss and delivers many health benefits, why not stick with it and make it your default diet? The less processed food you eat, the more chances you'll need to experience the health benefits from your hotel plan, so you don't need to see a doctor as often.

Natural ingredients have tons of vitamins and minerals. They need a high nutritional value. Coincidence or not, sirtuins can mostly be found in such ingredients (virtually fruits and veggies). Therefore, you'll get to unleash these benefits on your body by consuming these unique ingredients on a day to day basis.

Sirtfoods Have Anti-Aging Effect

Anti-aging is somehow linked to autophagy, an intracellular process of repairing or replacing damaged cell parts. Often this is rejuvenation at an intracellular level. We can't mention autophagy without a minimum of saying something about AMPK (adenosine monophosphate-activated protein kinase), an enzyme vital for cellular energy homeostasis. Therefore, this enzyme boosts energy by activating carboxylic acid, glucose, and oxidation when cellular energy is low. It represents the body's response when facing an elevated energy demand (e.g., an intense physical exercise).

However, a part of this response is that the lysosomal degradation pathway autophagy. Now you're probably wondering what sirtuins need to do with all of those. Well, SIRT1 can activate AMPK (and the opposite way around), so it is often considered one of the triggers of autophagy. But I'm getting to spare you all the chemical details that you simply can't remember. You should understand that autophagy rejuvenates the cell, and this process can happen to all of the cells in your body—ranging from those of your internal organs to those of your skin.

There are a couple of ways to induce autophagy, and it has a very positive effect on your health and overall lifespan. Just consider the cell as a car, and autophagy is when the skilled mechanic fixes or replaces any broken parts. The section will have an extended life, and this extrapolates to your overall experience. If your cells are functioning correctly, sort of a Swiss mechanical clock, then you'll expect increased longevity. You can't reverse aging, as there's no cure for it, and autophagy isn't "the fountain of youth." However, this process can significantly hamper aging and its effect. And therefore, the better part is that sirtuins, especially SIRT1, often activate it.

So far, people weren't conscious of too many ways to trigger autophagy. A number of them were doing it the hard way through intermittent fasting. Others were trying to induce it through an LCHF diet, just like the keto diet. Well, now there's an additional thanks to activating it, which is through the sirtfood diet.

Pros and Cons of Sirtfood Diet

Pros:

— The 'sirt foods' trigger the sirtuin in your body. (A kind of protein that helps shield your cells from dying and contracting diseases and controlling your body's metabolism.)

— In an experiment of 40 gym goers, each person lost on the average 7lb in a week without losing muscle mass.

— You can eat low amounts of chocolate and wine without you being affected.

— It contains foods that are primarily healthy and nourishing, like blueberries, walnuts, and tea.

— It is a long term health strategy that also reduces the aging process.

Cons:

There's a calorie reduction for the first week, which would make most people lose weight, irrespective of what food is consumed. Also, for the first three days, you eat 1,000 calories daily, and for the next four days you eat over 1,500 calories per day.

Intensively reducing your calorie intake is often harmful if your body isn't used to it and may cause you to be sluggish.

There is not enough proof that it follows through on its promises, most significantly the aspect of speeding from your metabolism.

You can only include foods on the sirtfood list examples are 'sirt juices,' soy, tea, and walnuts.

Concluding, the need of having a range of foods in your diet is reduced. You will look and feel good. For example, eating fruit and vegetables a day provides enough minerals and vitamins in your meals.

Is a Sirtfood Diet Really Effective?

There are no evident sign that the Sirtfood diet causes increased weight loss than a calorie-restricted diet regime.

Although various foods have beneficial properties, there are yet to be any long-term human studies to determine if eating a diet filled with sirtfoods has any concrete health benefits.

Nonetheless, the Sirtfood Diet publication's pilot study's outcomes were as follows:

After one week of following the diet and working out each day, the participants lost almost 5 pounds (3.2 kg) and claimed that they even gained some muscle tissue.

Yet, these outcomes are hardly surprising. Restricting your calorie intake to 1000 calories while exercising throughout the same period will almost always trigger weight loss.

This sort of fast fat reduction is not suitable for the long-term.

When your body is energy-deprived, it uses your emergency energy stores of glycogen while burning muscle and fat.

Each molecule of glycogen necessitates 3-4 atoms of water. Whenever your body uses glycogen, it removes water.

In the first week of an extreme calorie deficit, almost one-fifth of these weight loss is from fat, whereas one other two-thirds stems from water, glycogen, and muscle.

When your calories increase, the body replenishes its glycogen stores and you regain the lost weight.

Unfortunately, such a calorie deficit can cause the body to scale back its metabolism, meaning you require fewer calories per day.

A diet may help you lose a few pounds initially but once you finish dieting you are likely to put on the lost weight.

Three weeks could be long enough to have some measurable long-term effects for preventing illness.

Alternatively, adding sirtfoods to a routine diet might just be an incredible idea in the long term. You could finish your diet and start eating sirtfoods today.

This diet might help you lose weight since it's low in carbs; however, the weight is extremely likely to be put back on when the diet ends. The diet plan needs to be long term to have a positive effect on your long term wellbeing.

What Does this Involve?

The Sirtfood Diet contains two stages. For the first few days, you will only drink three 'sirt juices' and have only one meal (A total of 1000 calories each day). Over the next four days, you're allowed two sirt juices alongside two meals per day (total of 1,500 calories per day). Then you advance to the much easier phase 2. One juice alongside three 'balanced' meals, daily.

Can It Be Successful for Fat Loss?

Now you ought to shed weight only because you're eating fewer calories, notably at phase one. You would possibly cut fat faster with this specific diet than with any 'aged calorie-restricted' plan, and also you'll feel fitter. The writers assert that this diet is 'scientifically proven to get and obviate 7lb in a week'...

Well, it's well worth noting that loads of dietary plans have just been tested on 40 healthy, highly motivated human guinea pigs in a high tech gym in London's Knightsbridge. The researchers lost a mean of 7lb per week while revealing increases in muscular density and energy. But as long as the calorie restrictions of the very first week, fat loss could simply be caused by the acute decrease in calories.

The verdict

Further studies are required to identify the long-term effect on waistlines and standard health and see if sirt dieters lose the pounds more efficiently than if they were on other diet plans. We don't yet precisely understand what, if any, impact the of introducing sirtfoods into our daily diet will do.

Anybody has the power to stick with the monotony of juices and limit themselves to a short list of foods. This diet will allow you to enjoy chocolate and wine, well, not mountains of it!

Cutting Calories Will Consistently Provide Results

In the short term, cutting calories is a highly effective method of reducing your body fat. Wine and chocolate aside, the list of foods is made up of foods that dietitians and nutritionists urge for Good health (think fresh fruit and veg!).

Whether or not It works nicely enough to permit it to face out aside from the tens of thousands of weight loss plans which have trodden this tired course before additionally remains to be viewed. Goggins and Matten will likely find yourself, bestselling diet writers. However, I assume the mega-bucks will indeed flow after the pharmaceutical industry manages to make sirtuin modulators, which we're ready to soda. Therefore, there'll be no requirement to down still another carrot smoothie.

Getting Started

Starting the Sirtfood diet is extremely easy. It just takes a bit of preparation. If you do not know what Kale is or where you'd find tea, you'll have a learning curve, albeit very small. There's little in the way of starting the Sirtfood diet.

Things to Do

Since you'll be preparing and cooking healthy foods, you'll want to do a couple of things the week you start:

— Clear your cabinets and refrigerator of foods that are unhealthy, which might tempt you. You furthermore may have a low-calorie intake at the beginning, and you are doing not want to be tempted into a fast fix, which will set you back. Albeit you'll have new recipes, you'll feel that your old comfort foods are more comfortable at the instant.

— Shop for all of the ingredients that you will need for the week. If you purchase what you'll need, it's more cost-effective. Also, once you see the recipes, you'll notice that many ingredients overlap. You'll get to understand your portions as you proceed with the diet, but a minimum of you'll have what you would like and save yourself some trips to the shop.

— Wash, dry, cut, and store all of the foods that you simply need; that way, you do them conveniently prepared once you need them. This fact may make a new diet seem less tedious.

One necessary kitchen tool that you simply will need apart from the particular foods may be a juicer. You'll need a juicer as soon as you begin the Sirtfood diet. Juicers are everywhere so that they are relatively easy to seek out, but the standard ranges broadly. This way is often where price, function, and convenience come into play. You'll attend a well-liked emporium. Otherwise, you can find them online. Once you recognize what you're going after, you'll go searching.

The juicer's quality will also determine the nutritional quality and sometimes the taste of your juice, which we'll explain a bit later. Just know that purchasing an inexpensive juicer could seem like a good idea now, but if you opt to upgrade later, you'll have spent extra money, and twice. If you purchase a simple juicer, consider it as an investment into your health. Many of us have spent money on a gym membership that went unused for quadruple the value of 1 juicer. A juicer won't attend waste.

So, since not all juicers are alike, allow us to list a couple of the features you simply want to look for.

Centrifugal juicers:

Centrifugal juicers do precisely that; they use force to spin the food (most like vegetables like carrots, cucumbers, or kale leaves) at high speeds to the sidewalls, where there are blades. The food is pushed through a sieve then you do your juice. You should drink this rather quickly, as you'll lose nutrients the longer it's exposed to air (which it already has done because it was spinning), and it oxidizes, also like a bit of warmth from the friction creates a loss of nutrients and enzymes. This way is often the entire reason you're juicing, so now is essential. You're also left with tons of solid but very wet pulp as a byproduct, which means there were tons of fibrous parts of the plants that the juicer couldn't handle. This fact is often also a missed opportunity for more nutrients. You'll also get tons of (warmish) foam at the highest, which some people don't like. It's quick, and it's easy; however, it's usually the most cost-effective of the juicer types. If you want to, it's better than not having one in the least, but you'll reap your rewards later if you invest.

Masticating juicers:

Masticating juicers also do what they assert they're. They masticate or chew the food, albeit more slowly than the opposite type, by pulling it through gears that extract the juice. The machine pushes the pulp out. You'd have less pulp with this machine afterward. There's also less oxidation, and thus, more nutrients. They can also handle other sorts of foods (which varies by make and model), but that's something you ought to consider. You'll get some foam with this also, but not as much. Again, these are costlier and should be checked out as you'd an investment that you simply wouldn't use and discard. If you would like it to last, and you would like to get the foremost from your juicing and take it seriously, you'll want to spend a bit extra money and obtain what you need.

Twin-gear/triturating juicers:

These geared juicers have gears that grind alongside millimeters of space left between to tear open foods and grind the plants with only a dehydrated pulp that's left. These are the foremost nutrient-efficient juicers on the market. They leave virtually no foam, and that they are nutrient-dense as they're not disturbing the inner plant cells with oxidation. You can always tell in the look (color) and taste (richer) than other juices. You'll use different attachments to make different foods with most brands also so that they are versatile. These are the very best pricing of most of the juicers generally, and there also are brand variations like the others.

Citrus Juicers

There also are juicers specifically for citrus fruits. These can range from hand-held, col-press juicers to small electric or automatic cold-press juicers. They too vary in quality and price,

You can do a bit of research on the juicers that you simply may have. It'll help engage you more in the process and the journey you're close to taking!

Storing Juices

The most nutrition from them immediately, you ought to drink them directly. If needed, you'll pre-juice, and put it in glass jelly, Mason jars. The wide mouth variety with the plastic lids is sweet, airtight, and non-corrosive.

You can chill your drinks for the day by resting them on ice packs in an insulated lunch tote or cooler. In extreme cases, you'll juice one to 3 days of them (it is suggested at the utmost for optimal freshness, although you'll push it further out.

You may also find something to stay the juice chilled even while you're drinking at home. You'll put a jar in the refrigerator just before prepping, and after your juice, pour it into one. You'll make it a daily ritual of sorts. Have "your glass" that you simply prepare a day. If you favor straws, you'll even buy yourself a pleasant, reusable glass straw. None of those things are necessary for the diet, but any juice just tastes such a lot better when it's not from plastic.

Tips to Help You Get Started

Drink your juices because the earlier meals in the day will help you. It's an excellent way to start your day for three reasons.

— It will offer you energy for breakfast and lunch especially. By not having to digest heavy foods, your body saves time and energy, usually spent moving things around to travel through all the laborious motions. You'll be bound to feel lighter and more energetic in this manner. You'll always change this pattern after the upkeep phase, but you'll find that you simply want to stay that schedule.

— Have fruits and vegetables before starchy or cooked meals, regardless of how healthy the ingredients, is the best way to choose your digestion. Fruits and vegetables digest sooner, and therefore they breakdown into the compounds that we will use more readily. Consider it as having your salad before your dinner. It works in the same way. The heavier foods, grains, oils, meats, etc., take longer to digest. If you eat these first, they're going to slow things down, which is where you do a backup of food wanting to be weakened. This fact is often also once you may end up with indigestion.

— Juices, especially green juices, contain phytochemicals that function as antioxidants and contribute to our energy and mood. You'll notice that you simply feel much differently after drinking a green juice than you'd if you had eggs and sausage. You'll want to make a food diary and note things like this!

Be prepared to regulate to having lighter breakfasts for a little while. Most frequently, we refill with high protein, carbohydrate, and high-calorie meals early in the day. We may feel that we didn't get enough to eat, which we aren't full of initially. Oddly because it sounds, we may even miss the action of chewing. Some people got to chew their food to know they had a filling meal. It's something automatic that we don't consider. Some also will miss that crunch like with toast. Just concentrate on the present, and know this is often normal, which it'll pass.

Activation of Sirtuins

Although our understanding of the precise functions of all the Sirtuins is minimal, studies show that activating them can have the following benefits:

— Switching on fat burning and protection from weight gain: Sirtuins do that by increasing the mitochondrion's functionality (which is involved in energy production) and sparking a change in your metabolism to interrupt down more fat cells.

— They are improving memory by protecting neurons from damage. Sirtuins also boost learning skills and memory through the enhancement of synaptic plasticity. Synaptic plasticity refers to synapses' power to weaken or strengthen with time, thanks to a decrease or increase in their activity. This way is often essential because memories are represented by a different interconnected network of synapses in the brain. Synaptic plasticity is a crucial neurochemical foundation of memory and learning.

— Slowing down the Ageing Process: Sirtuins act as cell guarding enzymes. Thus, they protect the cells and hamper their aging process.

— Repairing cells: The Sirtuins repair cells damaged by re-activating cell functionality.

— Protection against diabetes: this happens through prevention against insulin resistance. Sirtuins do that by controlling blood glucose levels because this diet involves moderate consumption of carbohydrates. These foods cause increases in blood glucose levels, hence the necessity to release insulin, and because the blood glucose levels increase significantly, there's got to produce more insulin. Over time, cells become immune to insulin; hence, the necessity to supply more insulin leads to insulin resistance.

— Fighting Cancers: The chemicals working as sirtuin activators affect the function of sirtuin in several cells, i.e., by switching it on when in normal cells and shutting it down in cancerous cells. This way encourages the death of cancerous cells.

— Fighting inflammation: Sirtuins have a strong antioxidant effect that has the facility to scale back oxidative stress. This fact has positive effects on heart health and cardiovascular protection.

Macronutrients and Micronutrients

The basis of the sirtuin diet is often explained in simple terms or complex ways. However, it's essential to know how and why it works so that you'll appreciate the worth of what you're doing. It's also necessary to understand why these sirtuin rich foods help you maintain fidelity to your diet plan. Otherwise, you'll toss stuff in your meal with less nutrition that might defeat the aim of designing for one rich in sirtuins. Most significantly, this is often not a dietary fad. As you'll see, there's much wisdom contained in how humans have used natural foods, even for medicinal purposes, over thousands of years.

To understand how the Sirtfood diet works and why these particular foods are necessary, we'll check out their physical body role.

Sirtuin activity was first researched in yeast, where a mutation caused an extension in the yeast's lifespan. Sirtuins were also shown to slow aging in laboratory mice, fruit flies, and nematodes. As Sirtuins' research proved to transfer to mammals, they were examined for their use in diet and slowing the aging process. The sirtuins in humans are different in the typing, but they essentially add equivalent ways and reasons.

There are seven "members" that structure the sirtuin family. It's believed that sirtuins play an enormous role in regulating specific cells' functions, including proliferation (reproduction and growth of cells), apoptosis (death of cells). They promote survival and resist stress to extend longevity.

They are also seen to dam neurodegeneration (loss of function of the brain's nerve cells). They conduct their housekeeping functions by cleaning out toxic proteins and supporting the brain's ability to vary and adapt to different conditions or recuperate (i.e., brain plasticity). As a part of this, they also help reduce chronic inflammation and reduce something called oxidative stress. Oxidative stress is when there are too many cells damaging free radicals circulating in the body, and therefore the body cannot catch up by combating them with antioxidants. These factors are associated with age-related illness and weight, which again brings us back to discussing how they work.

You will see labels in Sirtuins that start with "SIR," representing "Silence Information Regulator" genes. They are doing precisely that, silence or regulate, as a part of their functions. The seven sirtuins humans work with are SIRT1, SIRT2, SIRT3, SIRT4, SIRT 5, SIRT6, and SIRT7. Each of those types is liable for different areas of protecting cells. They work by either stimulating or turning on certain gene expressions or reducing and turning off other gene expressions. This fact essentially means they will influence genes to do more or less of something, most of which they're already programmed to do.

Through enzyme reactions, each of the SIRT types affects different areas of cells that are liable for the metabolic processes that help take care of life. This way is often also associated with what organs and functions they're going to affect.

For example, the SIRT6 causes a gene expression in humans that affects striated muscle, fat tissue, brain, and heart. SIRT 3 would induce an expression of genes that affect the kidneys, liver, mind, and heart.

If we tie these concepts together, you'll see that the Sirtuin proteins can change the expression of genes, and in the case of the Sirtfood Diet, we care about how sirtuins can close up those genes are liable for speeding up aging and for weight management.

The other aspect of sirtuins' current conversation is that the function and, therefore, the power of calorie restriction on the physical body. Calorie restriction is just eating fewer calories. This fact, including exercise and reducing stress, is typically a mixture for weight loss. Calorie restriction has also proven across much research in animals and humans to extend one's lifespan.

We can look further at the role of sirtuins with calorie restriction and using the SIRT3 protein, which features a metabolism and aging function. Among all of the protein's consequences on the organic phenomenon (such as preventing cells from dying, reducing tumors from growing, etc.), we would like to know the effects of SIRT3 on weight for this book's aim.

The SIRT3 has high expression in those metabolically active tissues, as we stated earlier, and its ability to precise itself increases with caloric restriction, fasting, and exercise. On the contrary, it'll express itself less when the body features a high fat, high calorie-riddled diet.

A previous couple of highlights of sirtuins are their role in regulating telomeres and reducing inflammation, which also helps with staving off disease and aging.

Telomeres are sequences of proteins at the ends of chromosomes. When cells divide, these get shorter. As we age, they get shorter, and other stressors to the body also will contribute to the present. Maintaining these longer telomeres is that the key to slower aging. Additionally, the right diet, alongside exercise and other variables, can lengthen telomeres. SIRT6 is one among the sirtuins that, if activated, can help with DNA damage, inflammation, and oxidative stress. SIRT1 also helps with inflammatory response cycles that are associated with many age-related diseases.

Calories restriction, as we mentioned earlier, can extend life to a point.

Like fasting, maybe a stressor, these factors will stimulate the SIRT3 proteins to kick in and protect the body from the stressors and excess free radicals. Again, the telomere length is also affected.

To sum up, all of this information also shows that, contrary to some people's beliefs, genetics, like "it is what it is" or "it is my fate because Uncle Joe has something..." through our own lifestyle choices. What we are exposed to, we will influence action and changes in our genes. This fact is often quite empowering thought, and yet one more reason you ought to be excited to possess a science-based diet like the Sirtfood diet is available to you.

Having laid this all out before you, you ought to be ready to appreciate how and why these miraculous compounds add your favor to stay you youthful, healthy, and lean. If they're working hard for you, don't you feel that you simply should do something too? Well, you can, which is what the remainder of this book will do for you.

Sirtuins are a family of proteins that control cellular health. Sirtuins hold a crucial role in maintaining cellular homeostasis. Homeostasis involves regulating the cell in balance condition.

How Sirtuins Regulate Cellular Health with NAD+

Let assume your body's cells are like an office. In the office, many individuals perform various tasks with a selected objective: stay profitable and achieve the organization's mission efficiently for as long as possible. Many pieces are working on multiple tasks in the cells with a selected goal: staying healthy and functioning efficiently for as long as possible. Precisely like a company's task change, thanks to various internal and external developments, so do priorities in the cells. Someone has to run the office, control what needs to be done when it should be executed, who's getting to roll in the hay and to modify the course.

An Organization, therefore the body system, cannot function without what we mentioned above. But levels of NAD+ reduces with age, the function of sirtuin also decreased with age, a bit like all a part of the physical body, it's not that easy. Sirtuins manage everything that happens in the body cells.

Sirtuins as a Protein

Sirtuins are a family of proteins that might sound like the dietary protein found in beans and other protein foods. But in this case, we're talking about molecules called proteins, which functions in the entire body's cells in numbers of instructions. Assume proteins because the departments at a corporation, as an illustration, specializes in its specific task while coordinating other department's tasks.

A popular protein found in the body is named "hemoglobin" it's a part of the globin family of proteins and liable for transporting oxygen throughout the vessel. The myoglobin is that the hemoglobin's support, they together structure the globin family. Your body has almost 60,000 families of proteins in several spots, and sirtuins are one of those families. While hemoglobin is one in a family of two proteins, sirtuins are a family of seven.

Out of the seven sirtuins in the body cell, three of them function in the mitochondria, three add the nucleus, and one among the seven functions in the cytoplasm, each plays a spread of roles. The most purpose of sirtuins is that they remove acetyl groups from other proteins.

Acetyl groups drive some specific reactions. They're particular tags on proteins that other proteins acknowledge while they react with them. If proteins are the departments of the cell and DNA is that the CEO, the acetyl groups are the status of every department. For instance, if a protein occurs, then the sirtuin can function alongside it to make something happen, even as the CEO can work with any head to perform any task.

Sirtuins work with acetyl groups by doing what's called deacetylation. This fact suggests they acknowledge acetyl's presence on a molecule then delete the acetyl, which ties up the molecule for its job. Another way that sirtuins function is by removing acetyl groups (deacetylating) biological proteins like histones. For example, sirtuins deacetylate histones, which are part of a reduced sort of DNA called chromatin. The histone may be an ample bulky protein that the DNA surrounds itself. Let assume it is a Christmas tree, and therefore the DNA strand is that the strand of lights. When the histones have acetyl, the chromatin is open or unroll.

This unrolled chromatin means the DNA is being transcribed, a crucial process. However, it doesn't get to remain to unroll, as it's likely to wreck in this position, almost just like the Christmas lights could get destroyed or the bulbs can get damaged when they're unwieldy or stays too long. When sirtuins deacetylate the histones, the chromatin is closed or tightly and correctly wound, meaning organic phenomenon is stopped or silenced.

Sirtuins are discovered for about 20 years, and their primary aim and role was found in the 1990s. Since then, researchers are interested in reviewing them, identifying their importance, and asking several questions on what else will be learned about them.

Exercise

The expression of sirtuin in the muscle is suffering from a workout that controls changes in the cellular antioxidant system, mitochondrial biogenesis, and oxidative metabolism.

Skeletal muscles aren't only involved effectively and movement but also engaged in endocrine activities by their ability to secrete cytokines and transcription factors into the bloodstream, thereby, controls the function of other organs. Furthermore, the striated muscle may be a metabolically active tissue that plays an essential role in maintaining the body's metabolism. The striated muscle contains about 40% of the whole weight. Therefore, the insulin-stimulated uptake of glucose and the main energy-consuming lipid catabolism is especially at this site. For the striated muscle, metabolic flexibility is essential to preserve physiological processes and metabolic homeostasis. It determines the power to modify from glucose to lipid oxidation. Advances in the understanding of the molecular mechanisms underlying striated muscle activity are a therapeutic benefit. Sirtuins' roles are widely investigated in the striated muscle concerning their role in controlling glucose and lipid metabolism, insulin functions and sensitivity, function, and mitochondrial biogenesis.

Cellular metabolic stress results from workouts, which affects the sirtuins. The foremost studies sirtuins with this respect are SIRT1 and SIRT3, SIRT1 localized in the nucleus while SIRT3, in the mitochondria. SIRT3 is more expressed in type I muscle cells. A search conducted showed that mouse striated muscle SIRT3 reacted to the six weeks of voluntary exercise dynamically to coordinate the downstream molecular response (Palacios et al., 2009). The result also showed that movement causes a rise in SIRT3 protein, CREB, coactivator one alpha, and citrate synthesis activity.

The downregulation of CREB, AMP-activated protein kinase (AMPK) phosphorylation, and therefore the mRNA of PGC-1α are all symptoms of SIRT3 knockout. Showing that for SIRT3 to hold out the biological signals effectively, these key cellular molecules are essential. Palacios et al. Discovered that SIRT3 responds to exercise dynamically to reinforce muscular energy homeostasis through AMPK and PGC-1α. [10]. Voluntary exercise causes a rise in the SIRT3 content of striated muscle. Muscle Immobility can, therefore, cause the downregulation of SIRT3.

Furthermore, SIRT1 protein content and PGC-1 in the muscle tends to extend with exercise. Bayod et al. (2012) reported that SIRT1 protein content, as PGC-1 in rat's muscle, increased after 36 weeks of treadmill training and side enhancement in antioxidant defenses. There's a rise in ATP demand during exercise, which successively results in increased NAD+ level and NAD+/NADH ratio. The result's a rise in the substrate for SIRT1 and SIRT3. SIRT3 is liable for the increased ATP production also as a discount in protein synthesis in the mitochondria. The ATP produced activates and deacetylases tricarboxylic acid (TCA) enzymes, electron transport chain, and β-oxidation, which maximizes the supply of reducing equivalents for ATP production. SIRT1, on the opposite hand, responds to exercise by contributing towards mitochondrial biogenesis via independent mechanism and PGC1α-dependent.

In summary, strenuous exercises activate SIRT1, which reinforces biogenesis and mitochondrial oxidative capacity. Then, having several sessions of training will start both SIRT1 and also SIRT3, which successively activates ATP production also because of the mitochondrial antioxidant function.

Sirt Boosters

Sirtuin activators boost your mitochondria's activity, a part of the biological cell that is liable for energy assembly. This way successively mirrors the energy-boosting effects, which also occur thanks to exercise and fasting. The sirtfood diet is assumed to start a process called adipogenesis, which prevents fat cells from duplicating – which should interest any potential dieter.

The exciting part is that sirtuin activators influence your genetics. The notion of the 'genetic' lottery is embedded in the public consciousness, but genes are more changeable than you would possibly think. You will not be ready to change your eye color or your height, but you'll activate or deactivate specific genes supported by environmental factors. This way is often called epigenetics, and it's a desirable field of study.

Tips for Fulfillment

Fat burning, increasing muscles, and better cellular fitness—these are the guaranteed results of the Sirtfood diet.

Being healthy and losing weight is an everyday choice. You do take those first baby steps and see how it can change you and your life.

If you would like to reap the fantastic results of Sirtfoods, here are a few suggested ways to jumpstart your diet:

— Safety first - Before starting any particular diet or regimen, consult your healthcare provider, especially if you have existing illnesses. This way may make sure that the diet won't sabotage any medications that you only could be taking or harm your health. Don't worry; the SirtFood diet is relatively safe.

— Knowledge is power - This diet remains brand new, but there's still a fair amount of data available and more upcoming since this diet is fast gaining popularity. Additionally, you'll also search the web for recipes, food alternatives, nutrient content, and more.

— Follow the rules - SirtFood is bound to bring results, if and as long as you carefully follow the diet guide and suggested food.

— Help yourself - apart from following what's allowed in the food program, and you'll start by eliminating processed and starchy food from your regular diet. Stop eating junk! This fact may mean the results of the SirtFood Diet.

— Start a physical activity - SirtFood diet can indeed burn those fats and build muscle, but I like to recommend that you simply start adding physical activities to your daily routine. A 30-minute walk each day would do wonders for your body and can also mean the results. Additionally, there are many beautiful effects when exercising, like preventing and combating health conditions, improving your mood, promoting better sleep, burning calories, supplying you with an energy boost, and more.

— Hit the supermarket - The SirtFood diet depends on certain foods. These foods were chosen due to their sirtuin-triggering ability. So, if you are doing not follow the list, well, you won't see results. Don't worry, because I will be able to be providing a list of suggested foods. And they are not any overly expensive sort of foods, and you'll find it readily available almost anywhere (you might even have already got some lurking in your fridge).

— Be ready with the initial "restrictions" if you would like to ascertain different results; you do to "sacrifice" a little to realize the full benefits of the SirtFood diet. But don't worry, the primary three days are only the toughest ones for this diet since there'll be calorie restrictions involved, but rest assured that it'll become more comfortable every day. Although for others who tried the diet, the conditions set wasn't that tough for them, the rationale is careful planning of meals. You'll not go hungry with this diet if you select wisely.

— Plan your meals - Whatever diet you'll get on, planning your meals may be a big help. Not only will it reduce the strain from dieting, but you'll also even have the prospect to weigh your choices and fill in your cupboard. For the primary phase of this diet, you do follow a calorie count. You'll be surprised that there are many filling dishes allowed with fewer calories and full of sirtuins.

— Involve a diet partner - This diet could also greatly benefit your family, partner, or friends (not just for overweight individuals), plus it's easier once you have an accountability partner to remind you, share recipes with or maybe cook dishes with.

— Document your progress - you'll start by taking "before" pictures and take necessary body measurements. You'll also keep a food diary so that you'll watch your food intake. Observe the changes in your body with hebdomadally or phase. You'll even have a group of goals to push you further to continue with the diet.

— Be kind to yourself - don't set too high expectations. Yes, some can quickly lose 7 pounds in a week, but remember that our bodies aren't all the same; and in fact, your level of commitment also will count. Other variables might be adding an exercise regimen in the diet plan, making the losing weight process faster.

Top Sirtfood to Settle On

With all of the science and theory established, here are the very best 20 foods with the highest amount of sirtuins:

— Bird's-eye chilli

— Buckwheat

— Capers

— Celery

— Cocoa

— Coffee

— Extra-virgin vegetable oil

— Green tea

— Kale

— Lovage

— Medjool dates

— Parsley

— Red chicory

— Red onion

— Red wine

— Rocket

— Soy

— Strawberries

— Turmeric

— Walnuts

These will make the idea of the Sirtfood diet. However, there also are numerous other recommended foods, which are healthy and contain high amounts of sirtuins.

How the Sirtfood Diet Works

The Sirtfood Diet contains two stages that span three weeks. From then on, you can hold on "sirtifying" your daily Diet by adding as many sirtfoods as you can.

The Special recipes for both of those stages are often located in the Sirtfood Diet publication, compiled by the diet founders. You'll need to catch on to stick to alongside the diet program.

The foods are crammed with sirtfoods; however, they do comprise other ingredients besides only the "high 20 sirtfoods."

The majority of the components and sirtfoods are a breeze to get.

But, three of those signature ingredients demanded both of these stages -- matcha tea extract powder, lovage, and buckwheat -- May be costly or challenging to get.

A big part of the diet plan is its green juice, which you need to produce for yourself a couple of times every day. You will need a Juicer (a blender won't work) and a kitchen, while the ingredients are all recorded by weight. The recipe is below:

Sirtfood Green Juice

- — 75 g (2.5 ounces) lettuce

- — 30 g (1 ounce) arugula (rocket)

- — 5 g parsley

- — Two celery sticks

- — 1 cm (0.5 in) ginger half per green apple half a lemon

- — half per teaspoon matcha tea

Juice ingredients apart from your tea, extract powder and lemon and put them in a glass. Juice the lemon by hand, then add either juice and tea powder in your juice.

Period One

The Very First Phase lasts seven days and involves calorie limitation and tons of green juice. It's meant to jumpstart your weight-loss reduction and promised to efficiently assist you to lose 5 pounds (3.2 kg) in 7 days.

In the first three days of period one, calories are confined to 1000 calories: your three green juices a day and something else. Daily, you will need to pick a recipe from the publication, which involve sirtfoods just like the most vital portion of the meal.

Meal Examples comprise miso-glazed lettuce, the sirtfood omelet, or maybe a shrimp stirfry with buckwheat noodles.

On days 4--7, phase one, calories are raised to 1,500. This way consists of two green juices a day and a couple of sirtfood-rich meals that you simply select from the publication.

Period Two

Period two Lasts for two or three weeks. Throughout this "care" period, you ought to gradually lose weight.

There is no particular calorie limit for this specific period. You eat three meals containing high amounts of sirtfoods as well as a green juice daily.

The meals should be chosen from the recipes included later in this book.

After the Diet

You should repeat these stages until you reach your desired weight.

You're encouraged to stay on "sirtifying" your daily diet even after completing the stated periods by incorporating sirtfoods consistently into meals.

There are a large range of Sirtfood recipes in Sirtfood Diet books. It's possible to incorporate sirtfoods into your existing diet plan or in recipes that you already use.

You are also invited to continue drinking the green juice daily.

This will make the Sirtfood Diet a life-style change instead of a standard onetime diet.

Is it Sustainable and Healthy?

Sirtfoods are almost all nutritious choices and may have additional health benefits due to their anti-inflammatory and anti-inflammatory properties.

Eating a small number of exceptionally well-balanced meals can't meet most of your body's nutritional needs.

The Sirtfood Diet is restrictive and can offer no apparent, exceptional health and fitness benefits over another diet plan.

Moreover, eating just 1000 calories is, on average, not recommended without oversight of a doctor. Eating 1,500 calories each day is just too restrictive for a lot of men and women.

The diet requires drinking up to 3 green juices a day. Albeit liquids can become quite an excellent supply of minerals and vitamins, they're also a supply of sugars. Additionally, they comprise of almost none of the nutritious fiber which whole vegetables and fruits do.

Furthermore, sipping juice throughout the whole afternoon may be a terrible idea for your blood sugar levels, as well as your teeth.

Particularly throughout the first week, as the diet is restricted in food choice and calorie intake, it may be deficient in protein, minerals and vitamins.

Because of the minimal-carb levels and restrictive food choices, this diet could be tricky to stick to for the whole three weeks.

The high upfront cost of the juicer along with the time needed to buy specific juice and meal ingredients may be enough to dishearten a lot of men and women.

We regularly determine the advantages of drinking tea extract, we have concluded that it provides a vast selection of practical benefits.

Drinking just one cup a day can allow you to experience these positive effects emotionally and physically. Below are a couple of the advantages of drinking tea extract.

— Tea extract helps the human brain

Individuals who study a lot should consider buying matcha tea extract and they'll discover that drinking tea daily permits them to work better and more efficiently.

— It calms your metabolism

People looking to lose weight frequently find small benefits in drinking tea extract as it calms your metabolism. This means that they're going to lose fat faster. It can make you diet healthier and more balanced so they will be in a position to burn calories and fat and reduce the additional weight they're attempting to cut.

— It can help fight off cancers

Tea is one of the many healthy meals and drinks that can help to prevent cancer. Polyphenols available in tea extract are traditionally considered to help prevent cancer growth and dispersing in your system.

It does so by preventing the cells from copying and growing as fast.

— It can reduce ageing of skin

If you're attempting to slow the ageing processor to make sure your face doesn't develop wrinkles as fast; tea extract could also be just the thing to assist you. It's crucial that you also drink water; also, if you want the skin to stay healthy daily, 23 glasses of tea extract can boost your general skin health.

— It boosts your immune system

In addition to keeping away cancer, tea comprises free radicals that help keep different diseases off. This includes diabetes, arthritis, as well as other bone-related disorders. To experience these effects, you should start drinking tea extract regularly.

— It reduces your cholesterol levels

When people get older, they whine about increased cholesterol levels. Doctors and other caregivers, in many cases, say that tea extract can assist with managing a healthy cholesterol level along with avoiding unhealthy foods and exercise regularly.

— Green tea enhances your memory

A few glasses of tea extract weekly could also be just the thing that you need to help the mind improve and recall things better. This helps at work while analyzing life but you can also impress people with how well you can remember modest information!

Sirtuins, Fasting, and Metabolic Activities

SIRT1, a bit like other SIRTUINS family, is protein NAD+ dependent deacetylases related to cellular metabolism. All sirtuins, including SIRT1 are important for sensing energy status and protecting against metabolic stress. They coordinate cellular response towards Caloric Restriction(CR) in an organism. SIRT1's diverse location allows cells to sense changes in energy levels anywhere in the mitochondria, nucleus, and cytoplasm. They are related to metabolic health through the deacetylation of several target proteins like the muscles, the liver, endothelium, the heart, and fat.

SIRT1, SIRT6, and SIRT7 are localized in the nucleus, where they participate in consumers' deacetylation to influence organic phenomenon epigenetically. SIRT2 is found in the cytosol, while SIRT3, SIRT4, and SIRT5 are located in the mitochondria where they regulate metabolic enzyme activities also as moderate oxidative stress.

SIRT1, as most studies with regards to metabolism, aid in mediating the physiological adaptation to diets. Several studies have shown the impact of sirtuins on Caloric Restriction. Sirtuins deacetylase nonhistone proteins outline pathways involved in metabolic adaptation when there are metabolic restrictions. Caloric Restriction, on the opposite hand, causes the induction of expression of SIRT1 in humans. Mutations that cause loss of function in some sirtuins genes can cause a discount in the outputs of caloric restrictions. Therefore, sirtuins have subsequent metabolic processes:

Regulation in the Liver

The Liver regulates the body's glucose homeostasis. During fasting or caloric restriction, glucose level becomes low, leading to a sudden shift in hepatic metabolism to glycogen breakdown and gluconeogenesis to take care of glucose supply as acetone body production to mediate the energy deficit. Also, during caloric restriction or fasting, there's muscle activation and liver oxidation of fatty acids produced during lipolysis in white fat. For this switch to occur, there are several transcription factors involved to adapt to energy deprivation. SIRT1 intervenes in the metabolic control to ascertain the energy deficit.

At the initial stage of the fasting, the post glycogen breakdown phase, the glucagon's assembly by the pancreatic alpha cells to active gluconeogenesis in the Liver through the cyclic amp response element-binding protein (CREB), and CREB regulated transcription coactivator 2 (CRTC2). The fasting gets prolonged, and the effect is canceled out and replaced by SIRT1 mediated CRTC2 deacetylase, leading to targeting the coactivator for ubiquitin/proteasome-mediated destruction.

SIRT1, on the other hand, initiates the subsequent stage of gluconeogenesis through acetylation and activation of peroxisome proliferator-activated receptor coactivator one alpha, which is that the coactivator necessary for forkhead box O1. Additionally, to the power of SIRT1 to support gluconeogenesis, coactivator one alpha is required during the required mitochondrial biogenesis for the liver to accommodate the reduction in energy status. SIRT1 also activates carboxylic acid oxidation through deacetylation and activation of the nuclear receptor to extend energy production. SIRT1, when involved in acetylation and repression of glycolytic enzymes like phosphoglycerate mutate 1, can cause shutting down of the assembly of energy through glycolysis. SIRT6, on the other hand, are often served as a co-repressor for hypoxia-inducible Factor 1 Alpha to repress glycolysis. Since SIRT1 can transcriptionally induce SIRT6, sirtuins can coordinate the duration of your time for every fasting phase.

Aside from glucose homeostasis, the Liver also overtakes in lipid and cholesterol homeostasis during fasting. When there are caloric restrictions, the synthesis of fat and cholesterol in the Liver is turned off, while lipolysis in the white fat commences. The SIRT1, upon fasting, causes acetylation of steroid regulatory element-binding protein (SREBP) and targets the protein to destroy the ubiquitin-professor system. The result's that fat cholesterol synthesis will repress. During the regulation of cholesterol homeostasis, SIRT1 regulates the oxysterol receptor, thereby assisting the reversal of cholesterol transport from peripheral tissue through upregulation of the oxysterol receptor target gene ATP-binding cassette transporter A1 (ABCA1).

Further modulation of the cholesterol regulatory loop can be achieved via steroid receptor, necessary for the biosynthesis of cholesterol catabolic and steroid pathways. SIRT6 also participates in regulating cholesterol levels by repressing the expression and post-translational cleavage of SREBP1/2 into the active make. Furthermore, in the circadian regulation of metabolism, SIRT1 participates through regulating the cellular circadian clock.

Mitochondrial SIRT3 is crucial in the oxidation of carboxylic acid in mitochondria. Fasting or caloric restrictions may result in up-regulation of activities and levels of SIRT3 to assist carboxylic acid oxidation through deacetylation of long-chain specific acyl-CoA dehydrogenase. SIRT3 also can cause activation of ketogenesis and, therefore, the urea cycle in the Liver.

SIRT1 also Add it in the metabolic regulation in the muscle and white fat. Fasting causes a rise in the level of SIRT1, resulting in deacetylation of coactivator one alpha, which successively causes genes liable for fat oxidation to get activated. The reduction in energy state also starts AMPK, which can activate the expression of coactivator one alpha. The combined effects of the two processes will produce increased mitochondrial biogenesis alongside carboxylic acid oxidation in the muscle.

Sirtuins and Exercise

The expression of sirtuin in the muscle is suffering from a workout that controls changes in the cellular antioxidant system, mitochondrial biogenesis, and oxidative metabolism.

Skeletal muscles aren't only involved in significant and movement and involved in endocrine activities by their ability to secrete cytokines and transcription factors into the bloodstream, thereby, controls the function of other organs. Furthermore, the striated muscle may be a metabolically active tissue that plays an essential role in maintaining the body's metabolism. The striated muscle contains about 40% of the whole weight. Therefore, the insulin-stimulated uptake of glucose and the main energy-consuming lipid catabolism is especially at this site. For the striated muscle, metabolic flexibility is essential to preserve physiological processes and metabolic homeostasis. It determines the power to modify from glucose to lipid oxidation. Advances in the understanding of the molecular mechanisms underlying striated muscle activity are a therapeutic benefit. Sirtuins' roles are widely investigated in the striated muscle regarding their role in controlling glucose and lipid metabolism, insulin functions and sensitivity as function, and mitochondrial biogenesis.

Cellular metabolic stress results from workouts, which affects the sirtuins. The foremost studies sirtuins with this respect are SIRT1 and SIRT3, SIRT1 localized in the nucleus while SIRT3, in the mitochondria. SIRT3 is more expressed in type I muscle cells. A search conducted showed that mouse striated muscle SIRT3 reacted to the six weeks of voluntary exercise dynamically to coordinate the downstream molecular response (Palacios et al., 2009). The result also showed that movement causes a rise in SIRT3 protein, CREB, coactivator one alpha, and citrate synthesis activity.

The downregulation of CREB, AMP-activated protein kinase (AMPK) phosphorylation, and therefore the mRNA of PGC-1α are all symptoms of SIRT3 knockout. Showing that for SIRT3 to hold out the biological signals effectively, these key cellular molecules are essential. Palacios et al. Discovered that SIRT3 responds to exercise dynamically to reinforce muscular energy homeostasis through AMPK and PGC-1α. [10]. Voluntary exercise causes a rise in the SIRT3 content of striated muscle. Muscle Immobility can, therefore, cause the downregulation of SIRT3.

Furthermore, SIRT1 protein content and PGC-1 in the muscle tends to extend with exercise. Bayod et al. (2012) reported that SIRT1 protein content, as PGC-1 in rat's muscle, increased after 36 weeks of treadmill training and side enhancement in antioxidant defenses. During exercise, there's a rise in ATP demand, which successively results in increased NAD+ level and NAD+/NADH ratio. The result's a rise in the substrate for SIRT1 and SIRT3. SIRT3 is liable for the increased ATP production also as a discount in protein synthesis in the mitochondria. The ATP produced activates and deacetylases tricarboxylic acid (TCA) enzymes, electron transport chain, and β-oxidation, which maximizes the supply of reducing equivalents for ATP production. SIRT1, on the opposite hand, responds to exercise by contributing towards mitochondrial biogenesis via independent mechanism and PGC1α-dependent.

In summary, strenuous exercises activate SIRT1, which reinforces biogenesis and mitochondrial oxidative capacity. Then, having several sessions of training will start both SIRT1 and also SIRT3, which successively activates ATP production also because of the mitochondrial antioxidant function.

Sirtuins and Cancer

Sirtuins have dual functions, a few different quite a cancer, tissue cell, and cancer-specific expression according to the Sirtuins sort. They need contradicting roles in cancer or tumorigenesis, which we'll be discussing below.

SIRT1

Several studies show a correlation between sirtuins and cancer, especially SIRT1. The SIRT1 Prototype may be a well-known and studied protocol of the SIRT family. SIRT1 controls the deacetylation of histone and methylation, deacetylating lysine 26 with histone H1 (H1-K26Ac), on histone H3, its deacetylase lysine 9 (H3-K9Ac), and on histone H4 its deacetylase lysine 16 (H4-K16Ac). It also causes deacetylation of several nonhistone proteins, including the FOXO family and KU70, which participate in cell cycle regulation, metabolism, and necrobiosis induction. SIRT1 is proven to possess dual functions in tumorigenesis. It can act as a tumor promoter by several deacetylating proteins involved in DNA damage repair or tumor suppressor processes; and the inactivation of specific pathways. SIRT1 initiates, promotes, and progresses several malignant tumors like prostatic adenocarcinoma, carcinoma, carcinoma, leukemia, carcinoma, melanoma, ovarian, and gastric cancer (Cafara et al., 2019). Deacetylates of STAT3 by SIRT1 through suppression of its inhibitory effect on gluconeogenesis can accelerate malignancy thanks to the activation of proteins needed for survival, downregulation of tumor suppressor genes conferment of drug resistance. SIRT1 enhances cell survival and cancer progression through the deacetylation of multiple substrates like FOXO1, P53, and KU70.

SIRT1 can act as a tumor suppressor when it directly interacts with and repressed oncogenes like c-MYC (Yuan et al., 2009). A study by Willing and Ahmad in 2015 showed that different cancers like bladder, glioma, prostate, and ovarian cancer show lower levels of SIRT1. SIRT1 has been shown to possess a tumor suppressor effect in triple-negative carcinoma cells by determining cell growth and a block of cancer proliferation and cell growth (Yi et al., 2013). the twin attributes of SIRT1 in cancer could also be due to the various role of SIRT1 then requires further investigation.

SIRT6

SIRT6 has low deacetylation and ADP-ribosylation activities. It exhibits deacetylase activity when myristoyl and palmitoyl groups are far away from lysine residues. The situation of SIRT6 is, especially in the nucleus. It binds and deacetylates nucleosomes, chromatin, and several other TFs. in the endoplasmic reticulum, SIRT6 is additionally localized. It may regulate tumor necrosis factor α when myristoyl groups are far away from lysines 19 and 20, leading to macrophages' secretion. The manor function that SIRT6 does is to regulate cellular homeostasis through regulating DNA-damage repair, metabolism, and telomere maintenance. SIRT6 actions correlate that of SIRT1, as discussed earlier. A bit like SIRT1, SIRT6 is often involved in either tumor progression or suppression, counting on the tissue context. Tumor suppression occurs in some cancer cells like carcinoma and HCCs by the decrease's expression level of SIRT6 also as blockage of glycolysis pathways. Conversely, the upregulation of SIRT6 at MENA and protein level in carcinoma, prostatic adenocarcinoma, melanoma, and non-melanoma carcinoma results in oncogenic role tumorigenesis.

SIRT7

SIRT7 controls ribosomal RNA expression and is localized in the nucleus, where it partakes in RNA polI activation. It's related to the seven cellular pathways that regulate metabolism control, stress response, genome stability, aging, transcription, tumorigenesis, and ribosome biogenesis. In tumorigenesis, SIRT7 has an oncogenic role through activation of cancer proliferation by deacetylating specific promoters of varied genes concerned with tumor suppression. The overexpression and upregulation of SIRT7 in some cancer like ovarian cancer, osteosarcoma, prostatic adenocarcinoma, carcinoma, colorectal cancer, and HCC are related to the advanced tumor stage. The oncogenic properties of SIRT7 may as a result of its interaction with P53.

SIRT2

In the mitotic process, differentiation, cell motility, oxidative metabolism, and necrobiosis, SIRT2 is involved. It's involved in α-tubulin deacetylates, resulting in the cytoskeletal organization. SIRT2 shows tumor suppressor activity also as oncogenic activity in tumorigenesis. This tumor suppressor activity has been the merchandise of the deacetylation of several proteins involved in biological processes like DNA damage, cell proliferation, and cell integrity (Huang et al., 2017). SIRT2 can act as both tumor suppressor and promoter. It can either be upregulated or downregulated to cause tumor promotion. Also, low expression of SIRT2 can cause oncogenic activities in some quite tumors. The upregulation of SIRT2 in HCC, leukemia, neuroblastoma, and carcinoma end in vascular invasion, cell proliferation, and tumor growth.

On the other hand, low expression of SIRT2 in some cancer cells can cause tumor suppression. In moderately differentiated grade 2 carcinoma, SIRT2 exerts tumor suppressor effect thanks to low expression and deregulation of the G2/M phase, which correlates with poor prognosis.

SIRT3

SIRT3 is the best-characterized mitochondrial SIRT, which answers stress conditions by translocating into the mitochondrial matrix after the activation of the proteolytic process. SIRT3 controls the acetylation of several proteins involved in regulating oxidative stress, mitochondrial metabolism, and ROS production. The acetylation results are apoptosis prevention, growth arrest, senescence, and promotion of neoplastic cell proliferation. Stress on cells results in damage to the mitochondria, which successfully reduces SIRT3 activity, which correlates with a discount in deacetylation and NAD/NADH ratio as growth arrest. The upregulation of SIRT3 expression has been evident to play some roles in cancer development also as progression. Such cancers include; colon, oral squamous, gastric, renal, esophageal cancer, and melanoma (Finley and Haigis, 2012). SIRT3 enhances proliferation through abrogation of the anti-proliferative activity of P53 in mitochondria In bladder carcinoma. It interacts with KU70 and alters the DNA repair pathway in cervical cancer. SIRT3 has shown dual function in tumorigenesis. Its deacetylating activity on mitochondrial proteins like IDH2, SOD2, and FOXO3a inhibits mitochondrial ROS production and enhances neoplastic cell proliferation.

SIRT4

SIRT4 lacks nicotinamide adenine dinucleotide-dependent deacetylase activity but takes part in metabolism and genome stability. It displays ADP-ribosylase activity and negatively regulates mitochondrial glutamine metabolism by inhibition of glutamate dehydrogenase activity. Its effects on glutamine metabolism cause the control of cell cycle progression and proliferation. The impact that's so vital for genomic integrity during DNA damage. SIRT4 features a tumor suppressor effect when it arrests the cell cycle and inhibits proliferation, invasion, and cell migration.

On the opposite hand, low expression of SIRT4 is present in some cancers like breast, colon, bladder, thyroid, stomach, and ovarian cancer and correlates with a worse prognosis. Loss of SIRT4 has been shown to cause stress-induced genomic instability and high glutamine-dependent proliferation resulting in a tumorigenic phenotype. Overexpression of SIRT4 in colorectal cancer suppresses malignancy by blockage of neoplastic cell proliferation through the E-cadherin association.

SIRT5

The role of SIRT5 in tumorigenesis isn't well specific but could be associated with a number of its activities like desuccinylation activity and induction of the antioxidant enzyme SOD1. High expression of SIRT5 can cause poor survival, increased drug resistance, and neoplastic cell growth.

Sirtfood Diet - Phase One

The Plan says that eating particular foods can trigger your "lean receptor" pathway which causes you to lose seven pounds in 7 days. Foods like ginseng, bittersweet chocolate, and milk contain a natural compound called polyphenols, which mimic fasting and exercise. Strawberries, red onions, cinnamon, and garlic are also powerful sirtfoods. These foods can activate the sirtuin pathway and cause weight loss.

The science seems appealing; however, there's little or no research to copy these claims. Plus, the guaranteed speed of weight reduction from the very first week is sort of quick and may not be in unison with the National Institute of Health's safe fat loss recommendations of a few pounds hebdomadally.

The Diet includes two stages:

Stage one endures for two days. For the initial three days, you simply drink three sirtfood green juices alongside a meal filled with sirtfoods for an overall total of 1000 calories. On days four through seven, you only drink a beverage, two juices, and a couple of meals, summing to 1,500 calories.

Stage 2 is a 14 day maintenance program, though it's created to shed weight steadily (perhaps not maintain your current weight). Daily meals should consist three balanced sirtfood meals plus one green juice.

After those three weeks, you're invited to keep on eating a diet filled with sirtfoods and drinking a green juice every day. It's possible to get several sirtfood cookbooks online and other recipes on the sirtfood *web site. One green juice recipe on the sirtfood web site is made up of a mixture of spinach and other leafy greens, celery, carrot, green apple, ginger, juice, and matcha. Buckwheat and lovage are also options to add into your own green juice. The diet urges that juices should be made in a juicer, not a blender, to taste better.

Now you will get to plan and access to the ingredients recommended to stick with this diet program properly. You'll need to invest in a good juicer, which won't set you back more than 100. Make free recipes that may be found later in this book.

The seasonality of ingredients such as kale and tomatoes can make it hard to buy these ingredients at certain times of the year. It's hard to follow the diet if you are travelling to social events or feeding a family with young children.

The diet cuts out numerous food varieties, such as limiting dairy foods that provide a range of crucial nutritional elements, including several that many parents lack. Excluding these from your diet is not an advocated strategy. What's more, the polyphenol-rich food matcha frequently contains lead from the tea leaves, which could be potentially dangerous for your health, particularly when consumed regularly. The diet includes a bitter and robust flavor, as does 85% black chocolate, which will even be suggested.

Sirtfood Nutrition Strategies

When choose to follow the Sirtfood daily Diet, you start with phase one — that lasts for two days. Throughout the first three days of this daily diet plan, you will drink three Sirtfood juices and also consume only one Sirtfood-rich meal, summing to a daily total of 1000 calories. In days four through seven, you will consume 1,500 calories daily, made up of two juices, and two healthy Sirtfood-rich meals. After that, Phase 1 is completed.

Phase 2 lasts a fortnight and enables one to eat three balanced Sirtfood-rich meals and one green juice every day. Once step 2 is finished, you revert back to a more ordinary eating manner; however; you are encouraged to incorporate sirtuin-activating foods into routine meal plans. It's possible to re-enter phases 1 and 2. After almost every cycle; you'll shed weight or excess fat.

Foods You'll Eat

You are advised to purchase a juicer once having decided that you are going to start the Sirtfood Diet. These foods and beverages are supported:

— green juices (including matcha tea extract, lovage, and buckwheat) tea Coffee

— Cocoa powder bittersweet chocolate

— Beef Kale

— Onions

— Parsley

— Coffee

— Copra oil

— Crimson

— chicory

— noodle

— berries

— Walnuts

— Eggs

— Bacon

— Turkey

— Sea-food

— Whole Grain pitas

— Cheese

— Hummus

— Buckwheat noodles Dark Wine

Can the Diet Function?

Phase 1's calorie deficit is the reason why you will lose a couple of pounds.

The reason for you not having lost weight is probably due to not having eaten enough sirtuin-activating foods to or having lowered your current calories consumed. Nearly all Sirtfoods are healthier and seem to reduce the risk of disease and help to maintain a healthy weight.

Preparing for the Initial Phase of this Daily Diet

The question is: Should sirtuins be game-changing?

Why aren't pharmaceutical and nutritional supplement organizations attempting to distill them into a tablet shape?

Short answer: The mechanics whereby they operate are still not fully known, meaning supplements won't necessarily be absorbed by your body due to the organic forms.

"In supplement type, it's poorly consumed by the whole human anatomy, however in its standard food matrix of wine, its bioavailability (just what proportion your physical body in a position to utilize is six-fold greater. We believe it's far better to eat up a vast selection of those nutritional elements from the type of pure whole foods, where they revolve alongside the countless additional natural bioactive plant compounds that act responsibly to reinforce our wellness."

Sirtfood Diet - Phase Two

Minerals and vitamins that women require supplements for contain iron, calcium, Vitamins B6, B12, and vitamin D. Men consume supplements of magnesium, fiber, Vitamins B9 vitamin C and E.

This premise pertains to weight loss diet plans too. Men and women's nutritional requirements impact weight loss and specific diet plans are tailored towards the individual genders.

Each diet plan and fat loss program and design has its own merits, and virtually most they work -- temporarily. Weight control and health care professionals assert nearly unanimously that the right blend of excellent nutrition and regular exercise is the perfect approach to lose weight and keep it off effortlessly.

This should not make it tough to lose or maintain a healthy weight for a normal person; however, the Sirtfood diet may help individuals struggling with the classic approach. However, I believe in blending the Sirtfood diet with exercise.

The Sirtdiet Basics

With an estimated 650 million obese adults internationally, it's vital that you simply encounter nutritious eating and workout regimes that will be attainable. The Sirtfood diet does only that. The notion is that food items are getting to occupy the skeletal gene's pathways that are sometimes actuated by exercise and fasting. The incredible thing is that food and beverage, like black chocolate and wine, also contain polyphenols that trigger the enzymes that mimic fasting and exercise.

Exercise Throughout the First Few Weeks

In the very first fourteen days of the dietary plan, where your calorie consumption is paid off, it would be sensible to discontinue or reduce exercise volume while the physical body adjusts to fewer calories. Listen to your own body and if you are feeling tired or consume less energy than usual, don't work out. As an alternate, make sure you remain centered on the basic pertinent to a wholesome lifestyle, like adding sufficient daily amounts of fiber, fruit and protein, and veggies.

When you do exercise, it's crucial to eat protein an hour afterwards. Protein fixes muscles after exercise, reduces soreness, and also may aid recovery. There are undoubtedly various recipes, including protein, that'll probably be perfect for post-exercise ingestion, just like the sirt chilli con Carne or perhaps the garlic poultry and tofu salad. If you want something lighter, try the sirt sour smoothie, then put in some protein powder for extra benefit. The shape of the workout you are doing would be down for you. However, activities in the home will make it possible for you to decide when to exercise, the kinds of exercises that suit you personally, and, therefore, are comfortable and short.

The Sirtfood diet is a superb means to change your diet plan, lose weight, and feel much healthier. The very first few weeks can challenge you; however, it's crucial that you simply assess which foods are best to eat and which delicious recipes suit you personally. Be kind to yourself in the very first few weeks while the body adjusts and requires action efficiently if you decide to accomplish it whatsoever. If you're already somebody who partakes in intense or moderate exercise; then it could be that you stay on as usual or manage your fitness regime to account for the shift in diet. A bit like with any diet and exercise varies, it's about the person and how much you will be ready to push yourself.

The Sirtfood Bird's-Eye Chillies comprise the many sirtuin-activating nutrition Luteolin and Myricetin.

Earth's Eye Chillies(sometimes referred to as 'Thai chillies') are among the absolute best 20 Sirtfoods and appearance frequently from the recipe segments (here and here) with this site. Suppose you are not used to hot food. In that case, it's advised that you simply begin with half a chilli amount mentioned in the recipe, additionally to deseeding the chillies. It's possible to regulate the spice to taste in your diet plan.

Chilli were found in America, and have been a part of this diet since 7500 BC. Explorer Columbus brought it back to Spain from the 15 century, and its farming spread quickly throughout the rest of the world. Its intense heat was created as a plant defense system to cause vexation and discourage predators from feasting about it. Yet, many individuals enjoy adding it to their eating routines.

There Are over 200 forms, colored from yellowish to green to reddish to dark, and ranging in heat from slightly hot into mouth-blisteringly hot.

Earth's - Eye Chillies boast far greater sirtuin-activating credentials than the milder regular chillies, which are also used in the recipes.

Earth's -Eye Chillies are famous for their weight loss qualities. They're ready to play an integral part in increasing your system's metabolism by boosting your body's temperature. A faster rate, good nourishment, and waste expulsion may reduce the chances of fat accumulation in your system.

The compound found in Bird's-Eye chilli, which causes the burning sensation, is known as Capsaicin. The impacts of the chemical may vary among humans. But most frequent is that of a burning sensation in the throat, mouth, and stomach upon intake.

Chillies also boost the flavors of various foods.

If you've started drinking tea, congratulations, you will start reaping the benefits of the additional ordinary sirtuins seen in tea extract.

You'll lose fat more readily, and experience a revitalized soul and luminous skin.

Why is Drinking Tea Extract Vital?

Green Tea is the sole supplier of a couple of the strongest sirtuin bioactive, catechin. Catechins are so potent that just a small volume, one small cup, activates metabolism and reduces oxidative stress.

— Appetite-suppressant

You truly see a decrease in the urge to eat after a cup or two of tea extract. You will discover that you simply never consider food between meals.

— A small supply of caffeine

A cup of tea extract contains a quarter of the caffeine you'd see in a cup of java or half the caffeine you'd see in a cup of tea. This caffeine is just enough to unite with the catechins to have an increased fat burning effect. This may be the simplest way to convert fat into muscle.

— **More energy**

Catechins provide you with a modest all-natural buzz, which makes starting your afternoon a bit simpler.

— **Cumulative effect**

The power of two cups of tea extract is far better than 1 cup and three cups are much better than two cups.

You can get up to four of your SIRT 5 each day out of drinking tea extract if you drink four cups.

— **Zero-calorie**

Green Tea is fat-free. It'll not require sugar sweetener and provides you energy without consuming calories.

Five Most Useful Sirtfoods For Good health

Here are our greatest five most useful Sirtfoods for good health.

Dark Chocolate

This yummy cure keeps the guts fit and modulates vital signs, and it is filled with antioxidants. Dark-chocolate spikes growing older, and combat free radicals. Additionally, it reinforces the body's immune mechanisms and wards away infections. Even the flavanols in chocolate can improve blood flow and reduce cognitive damage.

Green Tea

Tea extract is probably one of the most effective all-natural remedies available on the market that is loaded with antioxidants and cancer-fighting chemicals. This drink is produced from the tea plant's dried leaves, which have been proven effective against pancreatic cancer, lung cancer, pancreatic cancer, diabetes, and prostate cancer. Green Tea reduces cardiovascular disease risk, lowers cholesterol, and protects against strokes. Its weight reduction benefits are copied by mathematics fiction.

Blueberries

Blueberries are an outstanding source of vitamin C, vitamin K, manganese, copper, and fiber. Additionally, they possess the best antioxidant content of most berries. These hot Sirtfoods boost resistance and neutralize the free radicals, which can damage cell structures. Low in carbs and calories, they're best for dieters. Recent studies imply that blueberries can help lessen abdominal fat and risk factors for metabolic syndrome. Filled with calcium, they additionally strengthen your muscles and protect against osteoporosis.

Capers

Capers boast strong anti-inflammatory effects, supplying a cocktail of vitamins, minerals, and antioxidants. They've just 2 3 calories per 100g and offer considerable amounts of potassium, calcium, vitamin K, riboflavin, iron, aluminum, and phytonutrients. Quercetin and rutin, the crucial antioxidants in capers, have potent analgesic, anti-bacterial, and anti-carcinogenic properties. Rutin helps treat and stop psoriasis, improves flow, and reduces harmful cholesterol levels in obese patients. Quercetin inhibits tumor development and also promotes immune function. The best way to use capers is usually by adding them to salads, pasta, pasta, and casseroles.

Turmeric

This spice was used in early times due to its curative properties. Curcumin, its ingredient, is a potent antioxidant and anti-inflammatory agent. This chemical reduces inflammation in the human body, helping prevent diabetes, chronic pain, cancer, obesity, cardiovascular problems, and various degenerative ailments. Turmeric also enriches your body's antioxidant capacity, struggles free deep damage, also improves brain functioning. This way is among only a few foods comprising BDNF (brain-derived neurotrophic factor), a protein that results in this growth, maturation, and survival of neural cells.

All of these are the five most useful Sirtfoods; however, there are quite a few different Sirtfoods with recognized health benefits, like apples, carrot, citrus, and pineapple. Redwine comprises sirtuin activators too. Your diet must also include vegetable oil, passionfruit, and onions that excite sirtuin cells and boost top antioxidant levels.

Grocery List for the Sirtfood Diet

All these are the highest-rated 20 foods to get a Sirtfood-rich diet program and ways to include them into your everyday meals.

- **Earth's** - Eye Chilli. Additionally, sold as Thai chillies, they are stronger than ordinary chillies and full of more nutritional elements. Utilize them to extend sour or sweet recipes.

- **Buckwheat**. Technically a pseudo-grain: it's a berry seed linked to rhubarb. Additionally, accessible noodle shape (like soba) makes sure that you're getting the wheat-free edition.

- **Capers**. If you're wondering, they're pickled flower buds. Sprinkle them a salad or roasted steaks.

- **Celery**. The leaves and hearts would be the significant healthful part, and thus don't throw them off if you're mixing a shakeup.

— **Chicory**. Red is most beneficial, but yellowish works too. Include it in a salad.

— **Cocoa**. The flavanol-rich type enhances vital signs, blood sugar cholesterol, and control. Search to get a high proportion of cacao.

— **Coffee**. Drink it shameful -- some signs can lower the absorption of sirtuin-activating nutritional elements.

— **Extra Virgin Steak Oil**. The extra-virgin type includes more Sirt benefits and also a much more pleasing flavor.

— **Green Tea or Matcha**. Add a bit of juice to boost the absorption of sirtuin-producing nutritional elements. Matcha is far better, but go Japanese, not Chinese, to steer beyond potential lead contamination.

— **Kale**. This vegetable includes vast levels of sirtuin-activating nutrition quercetin and kaempferol. Scrub it with copra oil and juice serve it as a salad.

— **Lovage.** It's an herb. Grow your personal onto a window sill and throw it into stirfries.

— **Medjool Dates.** However carefully, they are a hefty 66 percent glucose, don't raise glucose levels, and even have been connected to reduced diabetes and disorder levels.

— **Parsley.** Quite only a garnish -- it's saturated in apigenin. Throw into a juice or smoothie for the full benefit. Chicory Red is most beneficial, but yellowish functions fine. Throw it in a salad.

— **Red Onion.** The reddish variety is healthier personally, and also sweet enough to eat raw. Stir it and put into a salad or eat it with a hamburger.

— **Red Wine.** You have been conscious of resveratrol: the great news is that it's heat-stable, which suggests it's possible to profit from cooking alongside it (in addition to glugging it directly). Pinot noir gets got the utmost content.

— **Rocket.** one of the very least interfered-with salad greens out there. Drizzle it with vegetable oil.

— **Soy.** Soybeans and miso are saturated in sirtuin activators. Include it in stirfries.

— **Strawberries.** Though they're sweet, they simply comprise 1tsp of sugar per 100g -- and Research suggests that they improve the power to manage carbonated carbohydrates.

— **Turmeric.** Evidence suggests the curcumin inside its anti-cancer properties. It's difficult for your physical body to assimilate alone; however, cooking it into fluid and including black pepper increases absorption.

— **Walnuts.** Filled with calories and fat but well recognized in lessening disorder. Mash them up with a skillet to get a sirt-flavored pesto.

Sirtfoods are the revolutionary way of triggering our sirtuin genes in the best way possible. These are miracle foods, mostly filled with specific all-natural plant compounds, called polyphenols, that possess the potential to trigger our sirtuin genes by changing them. Essentially, they mimic the results of exercise and fasting. Doing this brings notable benefits by helping the system raise and control glucose levels, burn fat, build muscle, promote memory and health.

Because they're stationary, plants have developed an incredibly complex stress-response system and produce antioxidants to assist them in conforming to their environment's challenges. Once we consume these plants, we eat up these polyphenol nourishment. Their effect is strong: they trigger our very own inborn stress-response pathways.

Even though All plants possess stress-response techniques, just certain ones have grown to make impressive levels of sirtuin-activating polyphenols. A lot of these plants are sirtfoods. Their discovery ensures that rather than strict fasting regimens or tough exercise apps; there's a radically new way to trigger your sirtuin genes: eating a healthy diet loaded with sirtfoods. On top of that, the dietary plan involves putting (sirt)foods on your plate, so not carrying off them.

Would You Eat Meat with Your Sirtfood Diet?

The answer is often yes. The diet is not just comprised of ingesting a healthy part of beef. It suggests that protein becomes an essential addition in a Sirtfood-based diet decided to reap the foremost benefit in maintaining metabolism and lessening the muscle imbalance common in many fat loss programs. It is not just a beef heavy diet (we remember the awful breath out of the Atkins diet). It's very vegetarian-friendly and caters to just about everyone, which is exactly what makes it sensible and an alternate.

Leucine Is an alkanoic amino acid found in protein that divides and truly enriches the action of Sirtfoods. This usually means the right solution to consuming Sirtfoods is by mixing them with chicken, beef, or an alternative supply of leucine like eggs or fish.

Poultry may be eaten as it is an excellent source of protein, B vitamins, potassium, and phosphorous. Also, red-meat is another superb source of iron, protein, calcium, and B-complex vitamin 12 and could be consumed on three occasions (750g raw weight) weekly.

Foods Saturated in sirtuins (proteins which regulate cellular and metabolic purpose) can play a part in increasing our wellbeing, reducing inflammation, and potentially helping weight loss too. In the case that you're worried that this diet will be miserably restrictive, you're in luck: those sirtuin-activating foods aren't merely filled with good for your polyphenols, but they're also diverse, flavorful, and could be incorporated into your diet in a range of creative ways.

Sirtuin activators and sirtfoods are new in the world of science of nutrition. Now a 'sirtfood' is a food packed in sirtuin activators. Vitamins were discovered over 100 decades back, antioxidants 50 decades ago, and sirtuin activators only over ten decades ago.

The 1st sirtuin activator to be understood and effective was resveratrol, found in the skin of red grapes (and that is the reason why wine is traditionally believed to keep you still healthy), pomegranates, and Japanese knotweed.

Additional Sirtuin activators soon followed, like catechins (seen in tea extract and also presumed to fight cancer cells) and epicatechins in chocolate (accountable for the health benefits of chocolates).

However, research took off once the pharmaceutical giant GlaxoSmithKline bought the rights to get artificial resveratrol variations for 462 million. It hastens trial, like a cancer treatment; however, the results weren't impressive. This season the organization announced it had ceased the research.

However, today, it seems that eating sirtfoods filled naturally with sirtuin activators might be described as a way healthier, much better -- and cheaper -- alternative for supplements. It had been considering as the most recent trial of sirtfoods and the sirtfood dietary plan. Present results imply that sirtfoods target the same precise path for reducing weight and staying fit as dietary restriction and workout.

Resveratrol, seen in wine might help counteract the unfavorable effect of elevated fat/high glucose diets-SirtFood Research.

Red Wine fans have a new cause to watch. Researchers have located a new wellness advantage of resveratrol that occurs naturally in blueberries, raspberries, mulberries, grape skins, and crimson wine. Resveratol is recognized as a sirtuin activator.

Even though analyzing the results of resveratrol from the diet rhesus monkeys," Dr. J.P. Hyatt, a professor at Georgetown University, alongside his group of investigators, found a resveratrol supplement could counteract the harmful effect of a superior fat/high sugar diet onto the thoracic muscles. In previous animal studies, resveratrol has been shown to enhance mice's lifetime and hamper the disorder's onset. In 1 study, it revealed aerobics mice's fed with a superior fat/high sugar-free diet plan.

Even though these outcomes are reassuring, there could also be a desire to eat a superior fat/high sugar and just incorporate a glass of wine or maybe a cup of fresh fruit into someone's daily diet. The investigators highlight that the worth of a wholesome diet cannot be overemphasized.

However, for once, there's a reason to have a glass of wine.

Breakfast Recipes

Mushroom Scrambled Eggs

Ingredients

— 2 tbsp

— 1 teaspoon ground garlic

— 1 teaspoon mild curry powder

— 20g lettuce, approximately sliced

— 1 teaspoon extra virgin olive oil

— 1/2 bird's eye peeled, thinly chopped

— A couple of mushrooms, finely chopped

— 5g parsley, finely chopped

— *optional* Insert a seed mix for a topper plus Some Rooster Sauce for taste

Guidelines

Mix the curry and garlic powder, then add just a little water until you achieve a light-weight glue.

Steam the lettuce for 2 or 3 minutes.

Heat the oil in a skillet over moderate heat and fry the chilli and mushrooms for two or three minutes till they've begun to melt and brown.

Insert the eggs and spice paste, cook over moderate heat, add the carrot, and cook over medium heat for an extra minute. In the end, put in the parsley, mix well, and serve.

Blue Hawaii Smoothie

Ingredients

— 2 tablespoons rings or approximately 4-5 balls

— 1/2 cup frozen tomatoes

— Two tbsp ground flaxseed

— ⅛ cup tender coconut (unsweetened, organic)

— a few walnuts

— 1/2 cup fat-free yogurt

— 5-6 ice cubes dab of water

Guidelines

Throw all of the ingredients together in a mixer and mix until smooth. You would possibly get to prevent and awaken to receive it combined smoothly or put in additional water.

Turkey Breakfast Sausages

Ingredients

- — 1 lb. extra lean ground turkey

- — 1 Tbsp EVOO, and a little more to dirt pan

- — 1 Tbsp fennel seeds

- — 2 teaspoon smoked paprika

- — 1 teaspoon red pepper flakes

- — 1 teaspoon peppermint

- — 1 teaspoon chicken seasoning

- — A couple of shredded cheddar cheese

- — A couple of chives, finely chopped

- — A few shakes of garlic and onion powder

- — Two spins of pepper and salt

Guidelines

Preheat the oven to 350F.

Utilize a little EVOO to dirt a miniature muffin pan.

Combine all ingredients and blend thoroughly.

Fill each pit on top of the pan, then cook for about 15-20 minutes. Each toaster differs; therefore, when the temperature of the muffin arrives at 165, then remove.

Banana Pecan Muffins

Ingredients

— 3 Tbsp butter softened

— 4 ripe bananas

— 1 Tbsp honey

— ⅛ cup OJ

— 1 teaspoon cinnamon

— 2 cups all-purpose pasta

— 2 capsules a couple of pecans, sliced

— 1 Tbsp vanilla

Guidelines

Preheat the oven to 180°C/350°F.

Lightly grease rock bottom and sides of the muffin tin, then dust with flour.

Dust the surfaces of the tin gently with flour, then tap to eradicate any excess.

Peel and insert the batter to a bowl, and with a fork, mash the carrots; therefore, you do get a mixture of chunky and smooth, then forgot.

Insert the fruit juice, melted butter, eggs, vanilla, and spices and stir to mix.

Roughly chop the pecans onto a cutting board when using, then fold throughout the combination.

Spoon at the batter 3/4 full and bake in the oven for about 40 minutes, or until golden and cooked through.

Banana and Blueberry Muffins - SRC

Ingredients

— 4 large ripe banana, peeled and mashed

— 3/4 cup of sugar

— 1 egg, lightly crushed

— 1/2 cup of butter, melted (and a little extra to dust the interiors of this muffin tin)

— 2 cups of blueberries (if they are frozen, do not defrost them. simply pop them into the batter suspended and)

— 1 teaspoon baking powder

— 1 teaspoon baking soda

— 1/2 teaspoon salt

— 1 cup of coconut bread

— 1/2 cup of flour (or 1-1; two cup bread)

— 1/2 cup applesauce

Guidelines

Add mashed banana to an outsized bowl.

Insert sugar & egg and blend well.

Add spread and strawberries.

Sift all the dry ingredients together, then add the dry ingredients into the wet mix and blend lightly.

Set into 12 greased muffin cups

Bake for 20-30min in 180C or 350 F.

Morning Meal Sausage Gravy

Ingredients

- — 1 lb. sausage

- — 2 cups 2 percent milk (complete is great also)

- — 1/4 cup entire wheat bread salt

- — and a lot of pepper to flavor

Guidelines

Cook sausage from skillet.

Add flour and blend; cook for a few minutes.

Insert two cups of milk.

Whisk while gravy thickens and bubbles.

Add pepper and salt and keep to taste until flawless.

Let stand a moment approximately to ditch and performance over several snacks.

Easy Egg-white Muffins

Ingredients

— 7 egg-whites

— 6 tbsp or two large egg whites

— turkey bacon or bacon sausage

— sharp cheddar cheese or gouda green berry discretionary

— lettuce and hot sauce, hummus, flaxseeds, etc.

Guidelines

Use microwavable safe container, then spray entirely to prevent the egg from adhering, then pour egg whites into the dish.

Lay turkey bacon or bacon sausage towel, then cook.

Subsequently, toast your muffin, if preferred.

Then put the egg dish in the microwave for a half-hour. Afterward, with a spoon or fork, immediately flip the egg in the container and cook for an additional half-hour.

While the dish remains hot, sprinkle some cheese while preparing sausage.

The secret is to get a paste of some kind between each coating to place up the sandwich together, i.e., a tiny bit of hummus or maybe cheese.

Sweet Potato Hash

Ingredients

- — 1 Sweet-potato

- — 1/2 red pepper, diced

- — 3 green onions, peppermint leftover turkey, then sliced into bits (optional)

- — 1 Tbsp of butter - perhaps a bit less (I never quantify) carrot powder - a few shakes

- — Pepper - only a small dab to get a bit of warmth

- — pepper and salt to flavor

- — cheddar cheese (optional)

Guidelines

Stab a sweet potato and microwave for five minutes.

Remove from microwave, peel the skin off, and foliage.

At a skillet, on medium-high warmth, place peppers and butter and sauté to get a couple of minutes.

Insert potato bits and keep sautéing.

While sauté, add sweeteners, leafy vegetables, and green onions.

Insert a dab of cheddar and Revel in!

Asparagus, Mushroom Artichoke Strata

Ingredients

- — 1 little loaf of sourdough bread

- — 4 challah rolls

- — 8 eggs

- — 2 cups of milk

- — 1 teaspoon salt

- — 1/4 teaspoon black pepper

- — 1 cup Fontina cheese, cut into small chunks

- — 1/2 cup shredded Parmesan cheese

— 1 Tbsp butter (I used jojoba)

— 1 teaspoon dried mustard

— 1/2 can of artichoke hearts, sliced

— 1 bunch green onions, grated

— 1 bunch asparagus, cut into 1-inch bits

— 1 10oz package of baby Bella (cremini) mushrooms, chopped

Guidelines

Clean mushrooms and slice and trim asparagus, and cut into 1-inch pieces. Reserve in a bowl and scatter 1/2 teaspoon salt mixture.

Drain and dice the artichoke hearts.

Melt butter in a pan over moderate heat, sauté the asparagus and mushrooms before the mushrooms start to brown, for about 10 minutes.

Blend the artichoke core pieces into a bowl with a mushroom/asparagus mix. Set aside.

Cut or split a small sourdough loaf into 1-inch bits. (My loaf was a bit too small, therefore that I used four challah rolls again)

Grease a 9x13 inch baking dish and generate a base coating of bread at the plate. Spread 1/2 cup of Fontina cheese bread, and disperse half vegetable mixture on the cheese at a layer.

Put a layer of those vegetables and bread and high employing a 1/2 cup of Fontina cheese.

Whisk together eggs, salt, milk, powdered mustard, pepper into a bowl, and then pour the egg mixture on the vegetables and bread.

Preheat oven to 375 degrees.

Eliminate the casserole from the fridge and let it thicken for half an hour.

Spread all the Parmesan cheese at a coating in the strata.

Bake in the preheated oven until a knife inserted near the border comes out clean, 40 to 45 minutes. Let stand 5 to 10 minutes before cutting into squares.

Egg White Veggie Wontons w/Fontina topped w/ crispy Prosciutto

Ingredients

- — 1 cup egg whites

- — butter

- — fontina cheese mixed

- — shredded cheddar cheese

- — broccoli

- — I utilized wheat

- — chopped bits tomatoes

- — diced salt and pepper

- — prosciutto - two pieces

Guidelines

Remove Won Ton wrappers out of the freezer.

Pre Heat oven to 350.

Spray miniature cupcake tin with cooking spray.

After wrappers begin to defrost, peel off them carefully - apart, one at a time, and press cupcake tin lightly. 5. I sliced the wrappers having a few spreads. (optional)

Set a piece of cheese in every bottom.

Satisfy desired lettuce - I used pre-cooked broccoli bits and diced tomatoes.

Pour egg whites all toppings.

Sprinkle each with a number of those shredded cheddar.

Cook for about a quarter-hour, but start watching them afterward 10 - whenever they poof up - assess them poking the center with a fork.

While eggs are cooking, spray a sheet of foil with cooking spray, put two pieces of prosciutto onto it, and then cook at precisely the same period because of the egg whites. After 8 minutes, then take and let sit once it cools it becomes crispy and chop and high eggs!

Crunchy and Chewy Granola

Ingredients

- — 2 1/4 cup old-style yogurt

- — 1 Tbsp flax seeds

- — 1/4 tsp kosher salt

- — 1/2 tsp cinnamon

- — 1/4 ground ginger

- — 1/2 cup honey

- — 2 tbsp packaged splendid brown-sugar

- — 3/4 cup ounces raw peppers

- — 1/2 cup sliced peppers

- — 1/2 cup golden raisins

- — 1/2 cup dried cranberries

- — 1 Tbsp vanilla sugar to earn put a used vanilla bean in a full sugar bowl and allow simmer for per month at icebox.

Guidelines

Pre Heat oven to 300.

Line baking sheet with parchment paper.

Mix 9 components together.

Insert 1 cup hot water, then mix alongside hands and spread into a skinny coating over a baking sheet.

Cook for an hour, stirring 2-3 times, before turning black gold brown.

Remove from the oven and let cool.

Serve with fruit and sprinkle with sugar.

Power Balls

Ingredients

- 1 cup old fashion ginger, dried (I've used apple cinnamon-flavored oats also)

- 1/4 cup quinoa cooked using 3/4 cup orange juice

- 1/4 cup shredded unsweetened coconut

- 1/3 cup dried cranberry/raisin blend

- 1/3 cup dark chocolate chips

- 1/4 cup slivered almonds

- 1 Tbsp reduced-fat peanut butter

Guidelines

Cook quinoa in fruit juice. Then bring back boil and simmer for about 1-2 minutes. Let cool.

Combine chilled quinoa and the remaining ingredients into a bowl.

With wet hands and mix ingredients and appear golden ball sized chunks.

Set in a Tupperware and put in the refrigerator for 2 hours until firm.

Cinnamon Crescent Rolls

Ingredients

- 2 cans refrigerated crescent rolls

- 1 stick butter, softened

- 1/2 cup brown or white sugar

- 1 tbsp cinnamon

- Glaze

- 1/2 cup powdered sugar

- 1 tsp vanilla

- 2 tbsp milk

Guidelines

Heat oven to 350°F.

In a small bowl, combine sugar, butter, and cinnamon; beat until smooth.

Separate dough into rectangles.

Then spread each rectangle about two tbsp cinnamon butter mix.

Roll-up starting at the broadest side, as you'll ordinarily do to crescent rolls. Firmly press ends to seal.

Put each cinnamon filled croissant on a parchment lineup baking sheet. *Be sure that you simply line the cooking utensil, or that you simply may make a mess after *

Bake from 10 to fifteen minutes or until golden brown.

In a small bowl, combine all glaze ingredients, adding enough milk for the desired drizzling consistency. Drizzle over hot rolls.

Fresh fruit Pizza

Ingredients

— 4 crescent rolls (Rolled-out and poked with a fork)

— Two spoonfuls of Cream-cheese

— 1 teaspoon of sugar

— 1 teaspoon Vanilla extract

— Handful berries - chopped (You Can use raspberry or blueberries)

— Sliced almonds

Guidelines

Place crescent rolls nonstick pan, then prick a couple of times with a fork. Cook at 375 for about 14 minutes. Let cool.

In a bowl, combine cream, Vanilla infusion & sugar stirring with a spoon.

Spread onto crescent rolls, then add almonds and fruit.

I sprinkled a little more sugar on top after!

Main Meals

The Bell Pepper Fiesta

Serving: 4

Preparation time: 10 minutes

Cook Time: nil

Ingredients:

- 2 tablespoons dill, chopped

- 1 yellow onion, chopped

- 1 pound multi-colored peppers, cut, halved, seeded, and cut into thin strips

- 3 tablespoons organic olive oil

- 2 ½ tablespoons white wine vinegar

- Black pepper to taste

Guidelines

Take a bowl and blend in sweet pepper, onion, dill, pepper, oil, vinegar, and toss well.

Divide between bowls and serve.

Enjoy!

Nutrition (Per Serving)

Calories: 120

Fat: 3g

Carbohydrates: 1g

Protein: 6g

Spiced Up Pumpkin Seeds Bowls

Serving: 4

Preparation time: 10 minutes

Cook Time: 20 minutes

Ingredients:

— ½ tablespoon chilli powder

— ½ teaspoon cayenne

— 2 cups pumpkin seeds

— 2 teaspoons lime juice

Guidelines

Spread pumpkin seeds over a lined baking sheet, add juice, cayenne, and chilli powder.

Toss well.

Preheat your oven to 275 degrees F.

Roast in your oven for 20 minutes and transfer to small bowls.

Serve and enjoy!

Nutrition (Per Serving)

Calories: 170

Fat: 3g

Carbohydrates: 10g

Protein: 6g

Mozzarella Cauliflower Bars

Serving: 4

Preparation time: 10 minutes

Cook Time: 40 minutes

Ingredients:

— 1 cauliflower head, riced

— 12 cup low-fat mozzarella cheese, shredded

— ¼ cup egg whites

— 1 teaspoon Italian dressing, low fat

— Pepper to taste

Guidelines

Spread cauliflower rice over a lined baking sheet.

Preheat your oven to 375 degrees F.

Roast for 20 minutes.

Transfer to a bowl and spread pepper, cheese, seasoning, egg whites, and mix well.

Spread in a rectangular pan and press.

Transfer to oven and cook for 20 minutes more.

Serve and enjoy!

Nutrition (Per Serving)

Calories: 140

Fat: 2g

Carbohydrates: 6g

Protein: 6g

Chicken curry with potatoes and kale

For four servings:

- 600g chicken breast, cut into pieces

- 4 tablespoons of extra virgin olive oil

- 3 tablespoons turmeric

- 2 red onions, sliced

- 2 red chillies, finely chopped

- 3 cloves of garlic, finely chopped

- 1 tablespoon freshly chopped ginger

- 1 tablespoon curry powder

- 1 tin of small tomatoes (400ml)

- 500ml chicken broth

- 200ml coconut milk

- 2 pieces cardamom

- 1 cinnamon stick

- 600g potatoes (mainly waxy)

— 10g parsley, chopped

— 175g kale, chopped

— 5g coriander, chopped

Guidelines

Marinate the chicken in a teaspoon of vegetable oil and a tablespoon of turmeric for about half-hour. Then fry in a high frypan at high heat for about 4 minutes. Remove from the pan and put aside.

Heat a tablespoon of oil in a pan with chilli, garlic, onion, and ginger. Cook everything over medium heat, then add the spices and a tablespoon of turmeric and cook for an additional two minutes, stirring occasionally. Add tomatoes, cook for a further two minutes until finally chicken broth, coconut milk, cardamom, and cinnamon stick are added. Cook for about 45 to an hour and add some broth if necessary.

In the meantime, preheat the oven to 425 °. Peel and chop the potatoes. Bring water to the boil, add the potatoes with turmeric and cook for five minutes. Then pour off the water and let it evaporate for about 10 minutes. Then spread vegetable oil alongside the potatoes on a baking tray and bake in the oven for a half-hour.

When the potatoes and curry are almost ready, add the coriander, kale, and chicken and cook for five minutes until the chicken is hot.

Add parsley to the potatoes and serve with the chicken curry.

Fruit Skewers & Strawberry Dip

Ingredients

- 150g (5oz) red grapes

- 1 pineapple, (approx. 2lb weight) peeled and diced

- 400g (14oz) strawberries

Serves 4

147 calories per serving

Guidelines

Place 100g (3½ oz) of the strawberries into a kitchen mixer and blend until smooth. Pour the sauce into a serving bowl. Skewer the grapes, pineapple chunks, and remaining strawberries onto skewers. Serve alongside the strawberry dip.

Choc Nut Truffles

Ingredients

- 150g (5oz) desiccated (shredded) coconut

- 50g (2oz) walnuts, chopped

- 25g (1oz) hazelnuts, chopped

- 4 Medjool dates

- 2 tablespoons 100% cocoa powder or cacao nibs

- 1 tablespoon coconut oil

Makes 8

236 calories per serving

Guidelines

Place all of the ingredients into a blender and process until smooth and creamy. Using a teaspoon, scoop the mixture into bite-size pieces, then roll it into balls.

Place them into small paper cases, cover them, and chill for 1 hour before serving.

No-Bake Strawberry Flapjacks

Ingredients

— 75g (3oz) porridge oats

— 125g (4oz) dates

— 50g (2oz) strawberries

— 50g (2oz) peanuts (unsalted)

— 50g (2oz) walnuts

— 1 tablespoon coconut oil

— 2 tablespoons 100% cocoa powder or cacao nibs

Makes 8 portions, 182 calories each

Guidelines

Place all of the ingredients into a blender and process until they become a soft consistency. Spread the mixture onto a baking sheet or small flat tin. Press the mixture down and smooth it out. Cut it into 8 pieces, able to serve. You'll add a sprinkling of chocolate to garnish if you would like.

Chocolate Balls

Ingredients

— 50g (2oz) peanut butter (or almond butter)

— 25g (1oz) cocoa powder

— 25g (1oz) desiccated (shredded) coconut

— 1 tablespoon honey

— 1 tablespoon cocoa powder for coating

Makes 6 balls

115 calories per serving

Guidelines

Place the ingredients into a bowl and blend. Employing a teaspoon, scoop out a bit of the mixture and shape it into a ball. Roll the ball in a little chocolate and put it aside. Repeat for the remaining mixture. The balls are often eaten immediately or stored in the fridge.

Warm Berries & Cream

Ingredients

- 250g (9oz) blueberries

- 250g (9oz) strawberries

- 100g (3½ oz) redcurrants

- 100g (3½ oz) blackberries

- 4 tablespoons fresh whipped cream

- 1 tablespoon honey

- Zest and juice of 1 orange

Serves 4

180 calories per serving

Guidelines

Place all of the berries into a pan alongside the honey and fruit juice. Gently heat the berries for around 5 minutes until warmed through. Serve the berries into bowls and add a dollop of topping on top. Alternatively, you'll top them off with fromage frais or yogurt.

Chocolate Fondue

Ingredients

- — 125g (4oz) dark chocolate (min 85% cocoa)

- — 300g (11oz) strawberries

- — 200g (7oz) cherries

- — 2 apples, peeled, cored, and sliced

- — 100mls (3½ fl oz) double cream (heavy cream)

Serves 4

352 calories per serving

Guidelines

Place the chocolate and cream into a fondue pot or saucepan and warm it until smooth and creamy. Serve in the fondue pot or transfer it to a serving bowl. Scatter the fruit on a dish able to be dipped into the chocolate.

Walnut & Date Loaf

Ingredients

- — 250g (9oz) self-rising flour

- — 125g (4oz) Medjool dates, chopped

- — 50g (2oz) walnuts, chopped

- — 250mls (8fl oz) milk

- — 3 eggs

- — 1 medium banana, mashed

- — 1 teaspoon baking soda

Serves 12

166 calories per serving

Guidelines

Sieve the bicarbonate of soda and flour into a bowl. Add in the banana, eggs, milk, and dates and mix all the ingredients thoroughly. Transfer the mixture to a lined loaf tin and smooth it out. Scatter the walnuts on top. Bake the loaf in the oven at 180C/360F for 45 minutes. Transfer it to a wire rack to chill before serving.

Chocolate Brownies

Ingredients

- — 200g (7oz) dark chocolate (min 85% cocoa)

- 200g (7oz) Medjool dates, stone removed

- 100g (3½oz) walnuts, chopped

- 3 eggs

- 25mls (1fl oz) melted coconut oil

- 2 teaspoons vanilla essence

- ½ teaspoon baking soda

Makes 14, 197 calories per serving

Guidelines

Place the dates, chocolate, eggs, copra oil, bicarbonate of soda, and vanilla essence into a kitchen appliance and blend until smooth. Stir the walnuts into the mixture. Pour the mixture into a shallow baking tray. Transfer to the oven and bake at 180C/350F for 25-30 minutes. Allow it to chill. Cut into pieces and serve.

Crème Brûlée

Ingredients

- 400g (14oz) strawberries

- 300g (11oz) plain low-fat yogurt

- 125g (4oz) Greek yogurt

- 100g (3½oz) brown sugar

- 1 teaspoon vanilla extract

Serves 4

213 calories per serving

Guidelines

Divide the strawberries between 4 ramekin dishes. in a bowl combine the plain yogurt with the vanilla. Spoon the mixture onto the strawberries. Scoop the Greek yogurt on top. Sprinkle the sugar into each ramekin dish, completely covering the top. Place the containers under a hot grill (broiler) for around 3 minutes or until the sugar has caramelized.

Pistachio Fudge

Ingredients

- 225g (8oz) Medjool dates

- 100g (3½ oz) pistachio nuts, shelled (or other nuts)

- 50g (2oz) desiccated (shredded) coconut

— 25g (1oz) oats

— 2 tablespoons water

Serves 10

162 calories per serving

Guidelines

Place the dates, nuts, coconut, oats, and water into a kitchen appliance and process until the ingredients are well mixed. Remove the mixture and roll it to 2cm (1 inch) thick. Cut it into ten pieces and serve.

Spiced Poached Apples

Ingredients

— 4 apples

— 2 tablespoons honey

— 4-star anise

— 2 cinnamon sticks

— 300mls (½ pint) green tea

Serves 4

99 calories per serving

Guidelines

Place the honey and tea into a saucepan and convey to the boil. Add the apples, star anise, and cinnamon.

Reduce the warmth and simmer gently for a quarter-hour. Serve the apples with a dollop of crème Fraiche or Greek yogurt.

Black Forest Smoothie

Ingredients

- 100g (3½oz) frozen cherries

- 25g (1oz) kale

- 1 Medjool date

- 1 tablespoon cocoa powder

- 2 teaspoons chia seeds

- 200mls (7fl oz) milk or soya milk

Serves 1

337 calories per serving

Guidelines

Place all the ingredients into a blender and process until smooth and creamy. Serve in a glass.

Creamy Coffee Smoothie

Ingredients

— 1 banana

— 1 teaspoon chia seeds

— 1 teaspoon coffee

— ½ avocado

— 120mls (4fl oz) water

Serves 1

239 calories per serving

Guidelines

Place all the ingredients into a kitchen appliance or blender and blitz until smooth. You can add a little crushed ice too. This recipe will also double as a breakfast smoothie.

Strawberry Buckwheat Tabbouleh

Ingredients

- — 50g buckwheat

- — 1 tablespoon turmeric

- — 80g avocado

- — 65g tomatoes

- — 20 g red onion

- — 25 g dates, pitted

- — 1 tablespoon capers

- — 30g parsley

- — 100g strawberries

- — 1 tablespoon of olive oil

- — Juice of 1/2 lemon

- — 30g rocket salad

Guidelines

Boil the buckwheat alongside turmeric and let it sit.

Finely chop the avocado, tomatoes, red onions, dates, capers, and parsley and blend with the cooled buckwheat. Cut the strawberries and mix with the other ingredient and season with oil and lemon juice. Serve on the rocket salad.

Chilli con carne

Ingredients

- — 1 red onion, chopped

- — 3 cloves of garlic, finely chopped

- — 2 Tai chillies, finely chopped

- — 1 tablespoon of olive oil

- — 1 tablespoon turmeric

- — 1 tablespoon cumin

- — 400g minced beef

- — 150ml red wine

- — 1 red pepper, seeded and diced

- — 2 cans of small tomatoes (400ml each)

- — 1 tablespoon of tomato paste

- 1 tablespoon cocoa powder (without sugar)

- 150g canned kidney beans, drained

- 300ml beef broth

- 5g coriander green, chopped

- 5g parsley, chopped

- 160g buckwheat

Guidelines

Sauté the onions, garlic, and chillies in vegetable oil in a high fry pan or a frying pan at medium heat. After three minutes, add cumin and turmeric and stir.

Then add the minced meat and fry until everything is brown. Add the wine, bring back the boil, and reduce by half.

Add the peppers, tomatoes, ingredient, cocoa, kidney beans, and stock, stir and cook for an hour. Add a little water or broth if the chilli is just too dry.

Cook buckwheat consistent with the instructions on the packet and serve sprinkled with the chillies and fresh herbs.

Pizza

For the dough

- — 7g dry yeast

- — 1 teaspoon brown sugar

- — 300ml water

- — 200g buckwheat flour

- — 200g wheat flour for pasta

- — 1 tablespoon of olive oil

Guidelines

Dissolve dry yeast and sugar in water and leave covered for a quarter-hour.

Then prepare the dough mix the flour, add the yeast with water and oil.

Preheat oven to 425 °.

Then knead the dough well again and make two pizzas, each 30 cm in diameter, floured the surface with a kitchen utensil. You can make a skinny pizza that covers an entire baking sheet.

Spread the pizza dough on a baking tray lined with baking paper.

For the sauce

- 1/2 red onion, finely chopped

- 1 clove of garlic, finely chopped

- 1 teaspoon of olive oil

- 1 teaspoon oregano, dried

- 2 tablespoons red wine

- 1 can of strained tomatoes (400ml)

- 1 pinch of brown sugar

- 5g basil leaves

- 1 can of strained tomatoes (400ml)

- 1 pinch of sugar

- 5g basil leaves

Guidelines

Fry the garlic, onion, and sugar with vegetable oil, add the wine and oregano, and cook briefly. Then add the tomatoes and cook on low heat for a half-hour. Then put aside and add the fresh basil leaves.

Pizza topping and baking

Spread the specified amount of spaghetti sauce on the dough - leave the sides as free as possible, don't spread too thickly.

Then add the specified ingredients, for instance:

sliced purple onion and grilled eggplant;

Or goat cheese and cherry tomatoes;

Or chicken breast (grilled), red onions, and olives;

Or kale, chorizo, and red onions.

Then bake for about 12 minutes and, if desired, sprinkle with rocket, pepper, and chilli flakes.

Shitake soup with tofu

Ingredients

— 10g dried Wakame algae (instant)

— 1-liter vegetable stock

— 200g shitake mushrooms, sliced

- — 120g miso paste

- — 400g natural tofu, cut into cubes

- — 2 spring onions

- — 1 red chilli, chopped

Guidelines

Bring the stock to boil, add the mushrooms, and cook for two minutes. In the meantime, dissolve the miso paste in a bowl with some warm stock, put it back to the pot alongside the tofu, don't let it boil anymore. Soak the Wakame as required (on the packet), add the spring onions and t'ai chi, and stir again and serve.

Chicken with walnut pesto and salad

- — 15g parsley

- — 15g walnuts

- — 15g Parmesan cheese

- — 1 tablespoon of extra virgin olive oil juice of half a lemon

— 50ml water

— 150g chicken breast fillet

— 20g red onions, cut into strips

— 1 teaspoon red wine vinegar

— 35g rocket salad

— 100g cherry tomatoes, halved

— 1 teaspoon balsamic vinegar

Guidelines

For the pesto, place parsley, walnuts, parmesan, olive oil, half the juice, and a little water in a blender and blend to a paste.

Marinate the chicken in a tablespoon of pesto and, therefore, the remaining juice for a minimum of half-hour.

Preheat oven to 400 °.

Marinate the onions in wine vinegar for 10 minutes, then drain the liquid.

Fry the chicken in a coated pan on each side at medium heat and place in the preheated oven for 12 minutes.

Remove the chicken from the oven, pour another tablespoon of pesto over it, and let it rest for five minutes.

Mix the rocket, tomatoes, onions, and balsamic vinegar, place the chicken on top and pour the pesto's remaining over it.

Buckwheat noodles with salmon and rocket

For four servings:

— 2 tablespoons of extra virgin olive oil

— 1 red onion, finely chopped

— 2 cloves of garlic, finely chopped

— 2 red chillies, finely chopped

— 150g cherry tomatoes, halved

— 100ml white wine

— 300g buckwheat noodles

— 250g smoked salmon

— 2 tablespoons of capers juice of half a lemon

— 60g rocket salad

— 10g parsley, chopped

Guidelines

Heat 1 teaspoon of the oil in a coated pan, add onions, garlic, chilli at medium temperature, and fry briefly. Then add the tomatoes and therefore the wine to the pan and permit the wine to scale back.

Cook the pasta consistent with the instructions.

In the meantime, cut the salmon into strips and when the pasta is prepared, add it to the pan alongside the capers, juice, capers rocket, remaining vegetable oil, and parsley and blend. Then serve.

Salad with salmon and caramelized chicory

For one serving: 10g parsley

— Juice of a quarter of a lemon

— 1 tablespoon capers extra virgin olive oil

- — 1/4 avocado sliced

- — 100g cherry tomatoes, halved

- — 20g red onions, sliced

- — 50g rocket salad

- — 5g celery leaves

- — 150g salmon fillet without skin

- — 2 teaspoons of brown sugar 1 chicory, halved lengthwise

Guidelines

Preheat oven to 425 °.

The dressing: Mix parsley, juice, capers, and a couple of teaspoons of vegetable oil in a blender to prepare the sauce.

Mix in a bowl avocado, tomato, purple onion, and celery green for the salad. Rub the salmon with a little oil and fry it briefly on each side in a coated pan. Then place in the oven for about five minutes.

Mix one teaspoon of vegetable oil with the sugar and rub it into the chicory's cut surfaces. Fry on medium heat for 3 minutes in a pan.

Mix the salad with the dressing and serve with salmon and chicory.

Turkey meatball skewers

For four servings:

- — 4 sticks of lemongrass

- — 400g minced turkey

- — 2 cloves of garlic, finely chopped

- — 1 egg

- — 1 red chilli, finely chopped

- — 2 tablespoons lime juice

- — 2 tablespoons chopped coriander

- — 1 teaspoon turmeric

- — Pepper

- — Clean lemongrass, cut in half lengthwise and wash.

Guidelines

Mix the meat with the egg, chilli, garlic, coriander, olive oil, juice, turmeric, and a little pepper. Make small balls.

Put the balls on the lemongrass skewer and grill them as you wish. Cook them in the oven or fry them in the pan until the balls are ready. Serve with a small salad.

Cod with vegetables

For one serving:

- 20g miso

- 1 tablespoon of mirin

- 2 tablespoons of olive oil

- 40g celery, sliced

- 1 garlic clove finely chopped

- 200g cod fillet without skin

- 1 chilli, finely chopped

- 1 teaspoon finely chopped ginger

- 60g green beans

- 20g red onion, sliced

- — 50g kale, coarsely chopped

- — 30g buckwheat

- — 1 teaspoon turmeric

- — 1 teaspoon sesame seeds

- — 5g parsley, roughly chopped

- — 1 tablespoon soy sauce

Guidelines

Mix miso, mirin, and a tablespoon of oil in a bowl, then marinate the cod for a minimum of half-hour.

Preheat the oven to 425 °, then bake the cod for 10 minutes.

In the meantime, heat the remaining oil in a large frypan. Sauté the onion in it, then add the celery, garlic, chilli, ginger, green beans, and kale. Fry until the kale is completed. If necessary, add some water to facilitate the cooking process.

Boil buckwheat with the turmeric consistent with the instructions in the package.

When the buckwheat is prepared, add sesame, parsley, and soy to the vegetables and serve the buckwheat with vegetables and fish.

Mushroom Courgetti & Lemon-Caper Pesto

Ingredients

— 4 courgettes (zucchinis)

— 10 oyster mushrooms, sliced

— 1 red onion, sliced

— 2 tablespoons olive oil

— 2 tablespoons lemon caper pesto (see recipe)

— 50g (2oz) rocket (arugula) leaves

Serves 4

127 calories per serving

Guidelines

Spiralize the courgettes into spaghetti. If you don't have a spiralizer, finely cut the vegetables lengthways into long 'spaghetti' strips. Heat the vegetable oil in a frypan, add the mushrooms and onions and cook for minutes. Add in the courgettes and, therefore, the pesto and cook for five minutes. Scatter the rocket (arugula) leaves onto plates and serve the courgettes on top.

Chicken Stir-Fry

Ingredients

— 150g (5oz) egg noodles

— 50g (2oz) cauliflower florets, roughly chopped

— 25g (1oz) kale, finely chopped

— 25g (1oz) mange tout

— 2 sticks of celery, finely chopped

— 2 chicken breasts

— 1 red pepper (bell pepper), chopped

— 1 clove of garlic

— 2 tablespoons soy sauce

— 100mls (3½ fl oz) chicken stock (broth)

— 1 tablespoon olive oil

Serves 2

566 calories per serving

Guidelines

Cook the noodles consistent with the instructions, then put aside and keep warm. Heat the oil in a wok or frypan and add in the garlic and chicken. Add in the kale, celery, cauliflower, red pepper (bell pepper), mange tout, and cook for 4 minutes. Pour in the chicken broth (broth) and soy and cook for 3 minutes or until the chicken is thoroughly cooked. Stir in the cooked noodles and serve.

Tuna With Lemon-Herb Dressing

Ingredients

- 4 tuna steaks

- 1 tablespoon olive oil

For the dressing:

- 25g (1oz) pitted green olives, chopped

- 2 tablespoons fresh parsley, chopped

- 1 tablespoon fresh basil, chopped

— 2 tablespoons olive oil

— Freshly squeezed juice of 1 lemon

Serves 4

241 calories per serving

Guidelines

Heat a tablespoon of vegetable oil in a griddle pan. Add the tuna steaks and cook on high heat for 2-3 minutes on all sides. Reduce the cooking time if you would like them rare. Place the ingredients for the dressing into a bowl and mix them well. Serve the tuna steaks with a dollop of dressing over them. Serve with a leafy rocket.

Kale, Apple & Fennel Soup

Ingredients

— 450g (1lb) kale, chopped

— 200g (7oz) fennel, chopped

— 2 apples, peeled, cored, and chopped

— 2 tablespoons fresh parsley, chopped

— 1 tablespoon olive oil

— Sea salt

— Freshly ground black pepper

Serves 4

99 calories per serving

Guidelines

Heat the oil in a saucepan, add the kale and fennel and cook for five minutes until the fennel has softened. Stir in the apples and parsley. Cover and bring it to a boil, and simmer for 10 minutes. Employing a hand blender or kitchen appliance, blitz until the soup is smooth. Season with salt and pepper.

Lentil Soup

Ingredients

— 175g (6oz) red lentils

— 1 red onion, chopped

— 1 clove of garlic, chopped

— 2 sticks of celery, chopped

— 2 carrots, chopped ½ birds-eye chilli

— 1 teaspoon ground cumin

— 1 teaspoon ground turmeric

— 1 teaspoon ground coriander (cilantro)

— 1200mls (2 pints) vegetable stock (broth)

— 2 tablespoons olive oil

— Sea salt

— Freshly ground black pepper

Serves 4

147 calories per serving

Guidelines

Heat the oil in a saucepan and add the onion and cook for five minutes. Add in the carrots, lentils, celery, chilli, coriander (cilantro), cumin, turmeric, and garlic, and cook for five minutes. Pour in the stock (broth), bring it to the boil, reduce the warmth and simmer for 45 minutes. Employing a hand blender or kitchen appliance, puree the soup until smooth. Season with salt and pepper. Serve.

Cauliflower & Walnut Soup

Ingredients

- — 450g (1lb) cauliflower, chopped

- — 8 walnut halves, chopped

- — 1 red onion, chopped

- — 900mls (1½ pints) vegetable stock (broth)

- — 100mls (3½ fl oz) double cream (heavy cream)

- — ½ teaspoon turmeric

- — 1 tablespoon olive oil

Serves 4

249 calories per serving

Guidelines

Heat the oil in a saucepan, add the cauliflower and purple onion and cook for 4 minutes, stirring continuously. Pour in the stock (broth), bring back the boil, and cook for a quarter-hour. Stir in the walnuts, cream cheese, and turmeric. Employing a kitchen appliance or hand blender, process the soup until smooth and creamy. Serve into bowls and cover with a sprinkling of chopped walnuts.

Celery & Blue Cheese Soup

Ingredients

- — 125g (4oz) blue cheese

- — 25g (1oz) butter

- — 1 head of celery (approx. 650g)

- — 1 red onion, chopped

- — 900mls (1½ pints) chicken stock (broth)

- — 150mls (5fl oz) single cream

Serves 4

312 calories per serving

Guidelines

Heat the butter in a saucepan, add the onion and celery and cook until the vegetables have softened. Pour in the stock, bring back the boil, then reduce the warmth and simmer for a quarter-hour. Pour in the cream and stir in the cheese until it's melted. Serve and eat immediately.

Spicy Squash Soup

Ingredients

- 150g (5oz) kale
- 1 butternut squash, peeled, de-seeded, and chopped
- 1 red onion, chopped
- 3 bird's-eye chillies, chopped
- 3 cloves of garlic
- 2 teaspoons turmeric
- 1 teaspoon ground ginger
- 600mls (1 pint) vegetable stock (broth)
- 2 tablespoons olive oil

Serves 4

128 calories per serving

Guidelines

Heat the vegetable oil in a saucepan, add the chopped butternut squash and onion and cook for six minutes until softened. Stir in the kale, garlic, chilli, turmeric, ginger, and cook for two minutes, stirring constantly. Pour in the vegetable stock (broth), bring it to boil, and cook for 20 minutes. Using a kitchen appliance or a hand blender process until smooth. Serve on its own or with a swirl of cream or crème Fraiche. Enjoy.

French Onion Soup

Ingredients

- 750g (1¾ lbs.) red onions, thinly sliced

- 50g (2oz) Cheddar cheese, grated (shredded)

- 12g (½ oz) butter

- 2 teaspoons flour

- 2 slices wholemeal bread

- 900mls (1½ pints) beef stock (broth)

- 1 tablespoon olive oil

Serves 4

228 calories per serving

Guidelines

Heat the butter and oil in a large pan. Add the onions and gently cook on a coffee heat for 25 minutes, stirring occasionally. Add in the flour and mix well. Pour in the stock (broth) and keep going. Bring back the boil, reduce the warmth and simmer for a half-hour. Cut the slices of bread into triangles, sprinkle with cheese and place them under a hot grill (broiler) until the cheese has melted. Serve the soup into bowls and add two triangles of cheesy toast on top. Enjoy.

Salads

Kale and Beef salad

Ingredients

- 250g (9oz) kale, finely chopped
- 50g (2oz) walnuts, chopped
- 75g (3oz) beef, crumbled
- 1 apple, peeled, cored, and sliced
- 4 Medjool dates, chopped
- For the Dressing
- 75g (3oz) cranberries
- ½ red onion, chopped
- 3 tablespoons olive oil
- 3 tablespoons water
- 2 teaspoons honey
- 1 tablespoon red wine vinegar
- Sea salt

Serves 4

342 calories per serving

Guidelines

Place the ingredients for the dressing into a kitchen appliance and process until smooth. If it seems too thick, add a little extra water if necessary. Place all the ingredients for the salad into a bowl. Pour on the dressing and toss the salad until it's well coated in the mixture.

Arugula salad

Ingredients

- 75g (3oz) fresh rocket (arugula) leaves

- 100g (3½ oz) strawberries, halved

- 8 walnut halves

- 2 tablespoons flaxseeds

Serves 2

268 calories per serving

Guidelines

Combine all the ingredients in a bowl, then divide them into two plates. For an additional Sirt food boost, you'll drizzle over some vegetable oil.

Tuna, Tomato, and Eggs Salad

— 100g red chicory

— 150g tuna flakes in brine, drained

— 100g cucumber

— 25g rocket

— 6 kalamata olives, pitted

— 2 hard-boiled eggs, peeled and quartered

— 2 tomatoes, chopped

— 2 tbsp fresh parsley, chopped

— 1 red onion, chopped

— 1 celery stalk, chopped

— 1 tbsp capers

— 2 tbsp garlic vinaigrette

Guidelines

Cut red chicory, cucumber in small pieces and combine in a bowl; add the rocket, olives, tomatoes, red onion, celery.

Season the salad with capers, parsley, and garlic vinaigrette. Put on top of the salad tuna and the eggs season with oil and enjoy it.

Crude Brownie Bites

All out Time: 5 minutes

Serves: 6

Ingredients:

- 2½ cups entire walnuts

- ¼ cup almonds

- 2½ cups Medjool dates

- 1 cup cacao powder

- 1 teaspoon vanilla concentrate

- ⅛-¼ teaspoon ocean salt

Guidelines

Put everything in a nourishment processor until considerably well mixed.

Make into balls and put on a baking sheet and freeze for a half-hour or refrigerate for two hours.

Serve.

Potato Salad

Potato Salad - New Sirtfood Recipes

Ingredients: (serves 2)

— 200g celery, generally slashed

— 100g apple, typically slashed

— 50g walnuts, generally slashed

— 1 little red onion, generally slashed

— 1 head of chicory, slashed

— 10g level parsley, slashed

— 1 tbsp escapades

— 10g lovage or celery leaves, typically slashed

— For the dressing:

— 1 tbsp additional virgin olive oil

— 1 tsp balsamic vinegar

— 1 teaspoon Dijon mustard

— Juice of a large portion of a lemon

Guidelines

Blend the celery, apple, walnuts, onion, parsley, escapades, and lavage/celery in a medium-sized plate of mixed greens bowl and blend. Make the dressing by whisking together the oil, vinegar, mustard, and juice. Drizzle over the dish of mixed greens, blend and serve!

Chargrilled Beef

Ingredients:

— 100g potatoes, stripped and cut into 2cm bones

— 1 tbsp additional virgin olive oil

— 5g parsley, finely hacked

— 50g red onion, cut into rings 50g kale, cut

— 1 garlic clove, finely hacked

— 120–150g x 3.5cm-thick meat filet steak or 2cm-thick sirloin steak

— 40ml red wine

— 150ml meat stock

— 1 tsp tomato purée

— 1 tsp cornflour, broke up in 1 tbsp water

Guidelines

Heat the oven to 220°C/gas 7.

Put the potatoes in a pot of boiling water, take back to the boil and cook for 4–5 minutes at that time channel. Put in a simmering tin with one teaspoon of the oil and dish in the hot stove for 35–45 minutes. Turn the potatoes like clockwork to ensure, in any event, cooking. For the purpose, when cooked, remove from the oven, sprinkle with the hacked parsley, and blend well.

Fry the onion in 1 teaspoon of the oil over medium heat for 5–7 minutes, until delicate and pleasantly caramelized. Keep warm. Steam the kale for 2–3 minutes at that time channel. Fry the garlic tenderly in ½ teaspoon of oil for one moment, until delicate yet not shaded. Include the kale and fry for an extra 1–2 minutes, until soft. Keep warm.

Heat an ovenproof skillet over high heat until smoking. Coat the meat in ½ a teaspoon of the oil and fry in the hot skillet over medium-high heat as indicated by how you wish your filet done. If you want your meat medium, it's smarter to burn the meat and afterward move the container to a stove set at 220°C/gas 7 and finish the cooking that path for the endorsed occasions.

Remove the meat from the dish and forgot to rest. Add the wine to the recent skillet to boost any meat buildup. Cook to reduce the wine considerably, until syrupy and with a concentrated flavor.

Include the stock and tomato purée to the steak container and convey to the boil that adds the cornflour glue to thicken your sauce, including it a bit directly until you do your ideal consistency. Mix in any of the juices from the refreshed steak and present with the broiled potatoes, kale, onion rings, and wine sauce.

New Saag Paneer

279 calories

3 of your SIRT 5 per day

Serves 2 • Ready in a short time

— 2 tsp rapeseed oil 200g paneer.

— Cut into 3D shapes

— Salt and crisply ground dark pepper

— 1 red onion, cleaved

— 1 little thumb (3 cm) new ginger, stripped and cut into matchsticks

— 1 clove garlic, stripped and daintily cut

— 1 green bean stew, deseeded and finely cut

— 100g cherry tomatoes, split

— 1/2 tsp ground coriander

— 1/2 tsp ground cumin

— 1/4 tsp ground turmeric

— 1/2 tsp gentle stew powder

— 1/2 tsp salt

— 100g new spinach leaves

— Little bunch (10g) parsley, cleaved

Guidelines

Heat the oil in a wide, lidded skillet over high heat. Season the paneer liberally with salt and pepper and hurl it into the dish. Fry for a few moments until brilliant, blending regularly. Remove from the plate with a spoon and put in a safe spot.

Reduce the warmth and add the onion. Fry for five minutes before having the ginger, garlic, and stew. Cook for an additional few minutes before fitting the cherry tomatoes. Put them on top of the dish and cook for an extra 5 minutes.

Add the flavors and salt; at that time, mix. Return the paneer to the dish and blend until covered. Add the spinach to the container alongside the parsley and coriander and put the cover on. Permit the spinach to reduce for 1-2 minutes; at that time, add into the dish. Serve directly.

Mocha Chocolate Mousse

Everybody appreciates chocolate mousse, and this one has a brilliant light and breezy surface. It is brisk and straightforward to make and is best served the day after it's made.

Serves 4–6

Ingredients:

— 250g dim chocolate (85% cocoa solids)

— 6 medium unfenced eggs, isolated

— 4 tbsp solid dark espresso

— 4 tbsp almond milk

— Chocolate espresso beans, to enrich

Guidelines

Soften the chocolate in a large bowl set over a skillet of delicately stewing water, ensuring the bowl's bottom doesn't touch the water. Remove the bowl from the warmth and leave the dissolved chocolate to chill.

When the softened chocolate is at the right temperature, race in the egg yolks one at a time so they overlap in the espresso and almond milk.

Utilizing a hand-held electric blender, whisk the egg whites until a firm pinnacle structure; at that time, blend several tablespoons into the chocolate blend.

Move the mousse to special glasses and smooth the surface. Spread with stick film and chill for 2 hours. Enliven with chocolate espresso beans before serving.

Buckwheat Superfood Muesli

Ingredients:

— 20g buckwheat pieces

— 10g buckwheat puffs

— 15g coconut pieces or parched coconut

— 40g Medjool dates, hollowed and cleaved

— 15g walnuts, cleaved

— 10g cocoa nibs

— 100g strawberries, hulled and cleaved

— 100g plain Greek yogurt (or veggie lover elective, for example, soy or coconut yogurt)

Guidelines

Blend everything of the above ingredients together (forget about the strawberries and yogurt if not serving straight away).

If you want to make this in bulk, set it up the previous night and just join the dry ingredients when serving. Store it in an impermeable holder. All you do to do the subsequent day is include the strawberries and yogurt, and it's ready.

Exquisite Turmeric Pancakes with Lemon Yogurt Sauce

Serves: 8 hotcakes

Ingredients:

For The Yogurt Sauce

- — 1 cup plain Greek yogurt

- — 1 garlic clove, minced

- — 1 to 2 tablespoons lemon juice (from 1 lemon), to taste

- — ¼ teaspoon ground turmeric

- — 10 crisp mint leaves, minced

- — 2 teaspoons lemon pizzazz (from 1 lemon)

For The Pancakes

- — 2 teaspoons ground turmeric

— 1½ teaspoons ground cumin

— 1 teaspoon salt

— 1 teaspoon ground coriander

— ½ teaspoon garlic powder

— ½ teaspoon naturally ground dark pepper

— 1 head broccoli, cut into florets

— 3 enormous eggs, gently beaten

— 2 tablespoons plain unsweetened almond milk

— 1 cup almond flour

— 4 teaspoons coconut oil

Guidelines

Make the yogurt sauce. Taste and luxuriate with more juice, if possible. Set aside or freeze until you are prepared to serve.

Put the broccoli in a nourishment processor and heartbeat until the florets are separated into little pieces. Move the broccoli to a huge bowl and add the eggs, almond milk, and almond flour. Mix in the flavor blend and consolidate well.

Heat 1 teaspoon of the copra oil in a nonstick dish over medium-low heat and empty ¼ cup player into the skillet.

Cook the hotcake until little air pockets start to point out superficially, and therefore the base is brilliant darker for 2 to three minutes. Flip and cook the hotcake for two to three minutes more. To stay warm, move the cooked pancakes to a stove safe dish and put in a 200°F oven.

Keep making the staying three hotcakes, utilizing the remainder of the oil and player.

Sirt Chilli Con Carne

Serves 4

- — 1 red onion, finely cleaved

- — 3 garlic cloves, finely cleaved

- — 2 10,000-foot chillies, finely hacked

- — 1 tbsp additional virgin olive oil

- — 1 tbsp ground cumin

- — 1 tbsp ground turmeric

— 400g lean minced hamburger (5 percent fat)

— 150ml red wine

— 1 red pepper, cored, seeds evacuated and cut into reduced down pieces

— 2x 400g tins cleaved tomatoes

— 1 tbsp tomato purée

— 1 tbsp cocoa powder

— 150g tinned kidney beans

— 300ml hamburger stock

— 5g coriander, cleaved

— 5g parsley, cleaved

— 160g buckwheat

Guidelines

Fry the onion, garlic, and bean stew in the oil over medium heat for 2-3 minutes; at that time, include the spices.

Include the minced hamburger and dark-colored over high heat. Include the wine and permit it to rise to reduce it considerably.

You may add a little water to accomplish a thick, clingy consistency. Just before serving, mix in the chopped herbs.

In the interim, cook the buckwheat as indicated by the bundle guidelines and present with the stew.

Chickpea, Quinoa, and Turmeric Curry Recipe

Serves 6

Ingredients:

— 500g new potatoes, split

— 3 garlic cloves, squashed

— 3 teaspoons ground turmeric

— 1 teaspoon ground coriander

— 1 teaspoon stew drops or powder

— 1 teaspoon ground ginger

— 400g container of coconut milk

— 1 tbsp tomato purée

— 400g container of slashed tomatoes

— Salt and pepper

— 180g quinoa

— 400g container of chickpeas, depleted and flushed

— 150g spinach

Guidelines

Put the potatoes in a dish of cold water and convey to the boil; at that time, allow them to cook for around 25 minutes until stick a blade through them. Channel them well.

Put the potatoes in a huge skillet and include the garlic, turmeric, coriander, bean stew, ginger, coconut milk, tomato purée, and tomatoes. Bring back the boil, season with salt and pepper; at that time, including the quinoa with a cup of simply boil water (300ml).

Diminish the warmth to a stew, place the highest on and permit to cook. Throughout the subsequent half-hour, blending at regular intervals approximately to make sure nothing adheres to the bottom. (This may be a significant long cooking time, yet this often is the extent quinoa takes to cook with all of those ingredients against simply in water). Halfway through cooking, include the chickpeas. When there are only 5 minutes left, include the spinach and blend it in until it withers. Once the quinoa has cooked and is cushioned, not crunchy, it's prepared.

If you want to add a little heat, add a cut red bean stew to the cooking curry when you add the other spices.

Snacks

Kale chips

Ingredients:

- — 1 large head of curly kale, wash, dry, and pulled from stem

- — 1 tbsp. extra virgin olive oil

- — Minced parsley

- — A squeeze of lemon juice

- — Cayenne pepper (just a pinch)

- — Dash of soy sauce

Guidelines

In a large bowl, rip the kale from the stem into palm-sized pieces. Sprinkle the minced parsley, olive oil, soy sauce, a squeeze of the juice, and a tiny pinch of the cayenne powder. Toss with a group of tongs or salad forks, and confirm to coat all of the leaves.

If you do a dehydrator, turn it on to 118 F, opened up the kale on a dehydrator sheet, and leave it there for about 2 hours.

If you're cooking them, place parchment paper on top of a cooking utensil. Lay the bed of kale and separate it a little to make sure the kale is evenly toasted. Cook for 10-15 minutes maximum at 250F.

Honey nuts

Ingredients

— 150g (5oz) walnuts

— 150g (5oz) pecan nuts

— 50g (2oz) softened butter

— 1 tablespoon honey

— ½ bird's-eye chilli, very finely chopped and de-seeded

Makes 20 servings, 126 calories per serving

Guidelines

Preheat the oven to 180C/360F. Combine the butter, honey, and chilli in a bowl, then add the nuts and stir them well.

Spread the nuts onto a lined baking sheet and roast them in the oven for 10 minutes, stirring once halfway through. Remove from the oven and permit them to chill before eating.

Tofu Guacamole

Ingredients

- 225g (8oz) silken tofu

- 3 avocados

- 2 tablespoon fresh coriander (cilantro) chopped

- 1 bird's-eye chilli

- Juice of 1 lime

Serves 6

162 calories per serving

Guidelines

Place all of the ingredients into a kitchen appliance and blend a soft chunky consistency. Serve with crudités.

Watermelon Juice

Serves 1

Ingredients

— 20g of young kale leaves

— 250g of watermelon chunks

— 4 mint leaves

— ½ cucumber

Guidelines

1. Remove the stalks from the kale and roughly chop it.

2. Peel the cucumber, if preferred, then halve it and seed it.

3. Place all ingredients in a blender or juicer and process until you achieve the desired consistency. Serve immediately.

Snack bites 120g walnuts

— 30g dark chocolate (85% cocoa) 250g dates

— 1 tablespoon pure cocoa powder

— 1 tablespoon turmeric

— 1 tablespoon of olive oil

— Contents of a vanilla pod or some vanilla flavoring

Guidelines

Coarsely crumble the chocolate and blend it with the walnuts in a kitchen appliance into a fine powder.

Then add the other ingredients and stir until you have a consistent dough. If necessary, add 1 to 2 tablespoons of water.

Make 15 pieces from the mixture and refrigerate in an airtight tin for a minimum of one hour.

The bites will last for a week in the refrigerator.

Choc Bites

Makes 15-20 bites

Ingredients

— 1-2 tablespoons of water

— 1 tablespoon of extra-virgin olive oil

— 1 tablespoon of ground turmeric

— 250g of Medjool dates- pitted

— 1 tablespoon of vanilla extract or scraped seeds of 1 vanilla pod

— 30g dark of chocolate (85% cocoa solids) broken into pieces or cocoa nibs

— 120g of walnuts

— 1 tablespoon of cocoa powder

Guidelines

Place the chocolate and walnuts in a kitchen appliance and run it until you get a fine powder. Add the other ingredients (except water) and process as ball forms.

Depending on its consistency, you may or may not add water (we don't want it to be too sticky).

Make bite-sized balls and place them in the refrigerator in an airtight container for about an hour before serving. You could roll the balls in some desiccated coconut or cocoa if desired. They will survive for a couple of weeks in the refrigerator.

Berries Banana Smoothie

Serves 2

Ingredients

— ½ cup of coconut milk

— 1½ cups of mixed berries (strawberries and blueberries)- could be frozen or fresh

— ¾ cup of water

— 4 ice cubes

— 1 tablespoon of molasses

— 1 banana

Guidelines

1. Place all the ingredients in a blender and blend until smooth.

2. Add water to the smoothie until you achieve your desired consistency, then serve.

Grape and Melon Smoothie

Serves 1

Ingredients

— 100g of cantaloupe melon

— 100g of red seedless grapes

— 30g of young spinach leaves, stalks removed

— ½ cucumber

Guidelines

1. Peel the cucumber, then cut it into half. Remove the seeds and chop them roughly.

2. Peel the cantaloupe, deseed it, and cut it into chunks.

3. Place all ingredients in a blender and blend until smooth.

Green Tea Smoothie

Serves 1

Ingredients

— 2 teaspoons of honey

— 250ml of milk

— 2 teaspoons of matcha green tea powder

— 6 ice cubes

— ½ teaspoon of vanilla bean paste (not extract) or a scrape of the seeds from the vanilla pod

— 2 ripe bananas

Guidelines

Place all the ingredients in a blender and run until you achieve the desired consistency.

Serve into two glasses and luxuriate in.

Juice and Cocktails

Sirtfood green juice

Ingredients:

— 2 large handfuls of kale

— 5 grams of parsley

— ½ green apple

— 2–3 large stalks green celery plus the leaves

— A large handful rocket (about 30 g)

— Juice of ½ lemon

— ½ level tsp matcha green tea

A tiny handful of lovage leaves (optional)

Guidelines

Simply mix all the greens—rocket, parsley, kale, and lovage employing a juicer, just fully juice them. Your target is to juice around 50ml of green vegetables.

The next step is to feature the green apple and, therefore, the celery.

Simply squeeze the lemon into the juice. Presumably, you'll have quite 250ml of liquid at this stage.

When ready, pour into a glass, and you'll now add your matcha tea powder. Stir and enjoy!

Berries juice

Ingredients

- A cup of strawberries

- A cup of blueberries

- 1 green apple

- 2 stalk parsley

- 50g celery

- ½ teaspoon of matcha green tea

- ½ lemon

Guidelines

Wash the vegetables and fruits, blend. Also, add tea leave it

Squeeze the juice into it

With a fine mesh, strain the liquid if you would like

Transfer to a cup and top with water if need be

Grapefruit blast

Ingredients

- — 1 grapefruit, peeled

- — 2 stalks of celery

- — 50g (2oz) kale

- — ½ teaspoon matcha powder

Serves 1

71 calories per serving

Guidelines

Place all the ingredients into a blender with enough water to hide them and blitz until smooth.

Blueberry blend

Serving 2 - Ready in 2 minutes.

Ingredients

- — 1 ripe banana.

- — 100g blueberries.

— 100g blackberries.

— 2 table spoon natural yogurt.

— 200ml milk.

Guidelines

Blend all the things required together until smooth. Serve in two glasses.

Sirt Energy Balls

20 balls

Ingredients

— 1 mug of mixed nuts (with plenty of walnuts)

— 7 Medjool dates

— 1 tablespoon of coconut oil

— 2 tablespoons of cocoa powder

— Zest of 1 orange (optional)

Guidelines

Start by placing the nuts in a kitchen appliance and grind them until almost powdered (more or less depending on how you wish your energy balls).

Add the Medjool dates, copra oil, cacao powder, and rerun the blender until thoroughly mixed. Place the blend in a refrigerator for half an hour, then shape them into balls. You'll add in the zest of an orange as you blend.

Kale and Blackcurrant Smoothie

Serves 1

Ingredients

— 1 cup of freshly made green tea

— 2 teaspoon of honey

— 10 baby kale leaves with the stalks removed

— 1 ripe banana

— 40g of blackcurrants

— 6 ice cubes

Guidelines

First, wash, then stalk the blackcurrants and place them in a blender.

Pour the honey into the tea until it fully dissolves, then adds this to the blender. Add the remainder of

the ingredients and run the blender until you get a
smooth mixture. Serve immediately.

Desserts

Yogurt nuts and berries

Ingredients

- — 100g (3½ oz) plain Greek yogurt

- — 50g (2oz) berries, chopped

- — 6 walnut halves, chopped

- — A sprinkling of cocoa powder

- — Serves 1 296 calories

Guidelines

Stir half of the chopped berries into the yogurt. Using a glass, place a layer of yogurt with a sprinkling of berries and walnuts, followed by another layer until you reach the top of the glass. Garnish with walnut pieces and a dusting of chocolate.

Sirt muesli

Number of serving: 2

Prep time: Prepare the night before.

Ingredients:

- 200g of strawberries, hulled and chopped
- 200g of plain Greek yogurt (soy or coconut yogurt for vegans)
- 30g of either coconut flakes or desiccated coconut
- 40g of buckwheat flakes
- 30g of walnuts, chopped
- 80g of Medjool dates, pitted and chopped
- 20g of cocoa nibs
- 20g of buckwheat puffs

Guidelines

Mix all the dry ingredients in a container and conserve it in a dark place. Leave until the next day.

Put yogurt and strawberries in a food processor and blend them.

In a bowl, put the muesli and add the strawberries and yogurt mix all together and serve.

Spiced poached apples

Ingredients

- — 4 apples

- — 2 tablespoons honey

- — 4-star anise

- — 2 cinnamon sticks

- — 300mls (½ pint) green tea

Serves 4

99 calories per serving

Guidelines

Place the honey and tea into a saucepan and bring to the boil. Add the apples, star anise, and cinnamon.

Reduce the warmth and simmer gently for a quarter-hour. Serve the apples with a dollop of crème Fraiche or Greek yogurt.

Sirt Chocolate brownies

Ingredients

- 200g (7oz) dark chocolate (min 85% cocoa)

- 200g (7oz) Medjool dates, stone removed

- 100g (3½oz) walnuts, chopped

- 3 eggs

- 25mls (1fl oz) melted coconut oil

- 2 teaspoons vanilla essence

- ½ teaspoon baking soda

Makes 14 197 calories per serving

Guidelines

Place the honey and tea into a saucepan and bring to the boil. Add the apples, star anise, and cinnamon.

Reduce the warmth and simmer gently for a quarter-hour. Serve the apples with a dollop of crème Fraiche or Greek yogurt.

Pistachio fudge

Ingredients

- — 225g (8oz) Medjool dates

- — 100g (3½ oz) pistachio nuts, shelled (or other nuts)

- — 50g (2oz) desiccated (shredded) coconut

- — 25g (1oz) oats

- — 2 tablespoons water

Serves 10

162 calories per serving

Guidelines

Place the dates, nuts, coconut, oats, and water into a kitchen appliance and process until the ingredients are well mixed. Remove the mixture and roll it to 2cm (1 inch) thick. Cut it into ten pieces and serve.

Conclusion

Thanks again for getting this precise guide – *"Sirtfood Diet."*

The Sirtfood Diet program is designed for weight loss as well as improve your metal and physical health.

The Plan suggests that eating particular foods can trigger your "lean receptor" pathway and help you to lose seven pounds in 7 days.

Foods like ginseng, bittersweet chocolate, and milk contain a natural compound called polyphenols, which mimic fasting and exercise.

Strawberries, red onions, cinnamon, and garlic are also powerful sirtfoods. These foods can activate the sirtuin pathway to activate weight reduction.

The endorsed nourishments in the Sirtfood Diet are low in calories and high in vitamins, which means it is perfect for weight reduction. If you are going to follow this diet, make sure to eat tons of protein and differentiate the nourishments you eat to avoid nutrienence inadequacies.

I hope this book helps you find an appropriate and effective diet regime to assist you in your weight loss journey.

www.ingramcontent.com/pod-product-compliance
Lightning Source LLC
Chambersburg PA
CBHW061752250726
48657CB00001B/88